Children as Fellow Citizens

participation and commitment

Micha de Winter

Radcliffe Medical Press
Oxford • New York

© 1997 Micha de Winter

Radcliffe Medical Press Ltd
18 Marcham Road, Abingdon, Oxon OX14 1AA, UK

Radcliffe Medical Press, Inc.
141 Fifth Avenue, New York, NY 10010, USA

British Library Cataloguing in Publication Data

A catalogue record for this book is available from the British Library.

ISBN 1 85775 179 5

Library of Congress Cataloging-in-Publication Data is available.

Translated by BSA Texts, © December 1995
Typeset by Marksbury Multimedia Ltd, Midsomer Norton, Bath, UK

Contents

Introduction

Calling the children together, complain to them or scold them, then exact their consent – that is not a meeting. Calling the children together, hold a speech, stir their emotions and then select a few who have to shoulder the duties and responsibilities – that is not a meeting... Noise, chaos, voting to have done with it – that is a parody of a meeting. A meeting should be businesslike, the children's remarks should be listened to attentively and with interest – without deception or emphasis – a decision should be postponed until the moment the educator has worked out a plan. Just as an educator does not know something, is unable to do something or considers it impossible, so children have a right not to know, not to be able or to consider something impossible. You have to work hard to communicate with children ...

(Janusz Korczak, How to love a child, 1920)

Children, the educationalist Lea Dasberg wrote in 1975, have long been raised by keeping them down. Ever since the Enlightenment, to protect them from the evil world of adults, they have been confined more and more to the glasshouse of a special youthland. In this land the child was to be free to express its distinct nature unhindered and was to find shelter from the perverting influences of the street, child labour, wars and loose morals. This shielding has undoubtedly had its merits. Child labour has indeed become an exception in the West, very young people are seldom sent to fight as soldiers, and numerous measures have been taken to protect them from maltreatment, abuse and neglect. Moreover the recognition of their distinct nature has partly made it possible for a great deal of knowledge on upbringing, education, the development and health of young people to become available. Many a Western country is apparently a child's paradise. The special attention and protection have their drawbacks, however. For a large part of their young life the new generation is excluded from all sorts of things that happen in the world around them. This in fact also applies to many adults, albeit that they can in principle take action by exercising their civil rights. For young people this exclusion appears to be generally accepted and even fervently advocated by many proponents of the youthland idea. Young people, after all, should be free from all the cares and conflicts that adults have; there will be plenty of time for those later! This is where there is a price to pay. The more young people find themselves in the position of social outsiders, the less reason they have to feel committed to society. The world 'happens' to young people, they are not adequately taught to come to grips with it. A few examples: there 'will be' a playground in the neighbourhood; an unused site 'is built on'; there 'is' a new traffic plan for the district; usually with public consultation, but not with young people. Pupils are talked with a lot in school, but their opinion on the way the school itself operates, where they spend so many hours of their lives; that question is hardly, if ever, asked. Finally, the youngster who finds himself involved in counselling to learn how to handle his problems better, often ends up in a situation which promotes rather than combats powerlessness.

In this way present-day children learn that their active commitment to, and joint responsibility for, their own living environment is not very much appreciated, just as many of their parents found. Society presents itself to them as an anonymous quantity. Who knows who the playgrounds in the neighbourhood belong to, who is responsible for maintenance and hygiene, whom to turn to to get something done about insecurity on the streets. And what child feels that the school is also his or hers, so that by breaking windows he is also breaking his own windows. This is what the world looks like to the present generation; however smart they are, they *do not count* until maturity. Then all of a sudden society expects responsibility, independence and, in particular, commitment. This miscalculation is the major theme of this book. The proposition is that all these necessary social qualities do not come automatically. Young people therefore should be taken by the hand in all those contexts in which they learn and live. Active participation is the key. This is a condition for beginning to feel committed to the various social circles they are part of. The rewards this may yield are not only in the future, but in the present as well. Every child, every young person, likes to be important, to be appreciated, to mean something in the community. To be allowed to take responsibility contributes to the creation of confidence, self-respect and a feeling of solidarity. This can be seen when young children in the family or in day-care enjoy being able to assist parents or teachers. It can also be observed in the enthusiasm with which primary school pupils apply themselves to projects in the neighbourhood. And it also holds good for somewhat older children, a group less often discussed in this book, that they are quite willing to bear responsibility, that they want to take a meaningful part in the context they are in. In the chapters that follow it will become clear that these apparently obvious things are not at all obvious in day-to-day practice.

The care of children in modern western societies is characterized by a peculiar paradox. Authorities, experts and media appear to be considerably more interested in children's health and their problems, the conditions in which they grow up and the perspectives they can be offered, than in the children themselves. Growth and development of children are monitored in a practically perfect way; their parents, if they so wish, receive ample professional support in care and education. And for each new intervention, a matching problem group can be found[1]. Notwithstanding this good individual preventive care we cannot in the least say that young people grow up in optimum circumstances. Because of the very fixation on individual health and well-being, numerous conditions influencing the quality of life (and eventually the health and development potential as well) of children and young people remain practically undiscussed. However much a Western country may seem to be a little paradise for children and young people, this should still be the subject of serious comment. We may wonder for instance, how child-friendly the physical environment is in which young people grow up; why there are considerable differences between young people from different socio-economic strata of the population; how much material, emotional and social space is available nowadays for young people to develop into independent, critical and responsible adults. Modern youth policy views children and young people mainly as objects of care. To a great extent, however, youth policy turns out to be *facilities policy*. Few local authorities appear to base their policy on an exchange of ideas with children and young people. This approach contrasts strangely with the principles stated in all sorts of official government documents. The increase of commitment to the personal living environment, for instance, is one of the principal pillars of the social renewal movements in European countries. The activation of the citizens' vital capabilities was one of the central ideas of the new Netherlands welfare policy in the nineties (Ministry of Welfare, Public Health and Cultural Affairs, 1991). The question, therefore, is why the voice of young people is heard so little in youth policy. Perhaps it is because adults think they know what the young want and what they need? Perhaps it is because it is so difficult to get into contact with them, or because it is so difficult to interest them in local policy, as many a local policy maker complains (Hazekamp *et al.*, 1993)? Many historical and present-day experiments are reviewed in this book, in which young people are directly involved in the realization of policy and facilities. By means of these examples the obvious conclusion forces itself upon us that a *dialogue* with young people is a basic condition for successful youth policy at a local level. But however obvious this conclusion may seem, practice proves that active involvement of children and young people in their own living environment is still hardly seen as an aim or as an instrument of youth policy.

It is therefore in the interest of the quality of the child's existence to re-assess the way in which society treats young people (cf. de Winter, 1990). In

---

[1]An example is the latest trend in schools to introduce testing for 'failure anxiety', aiming to detect the group of pupils with examination fear as early as possible. Such an approach raises difficulties at school to the level of an individual psychological syndrome. In this way the influence of the 'performance race', which is socially construed and which gets many pupils into difficulties, remains out of sight (cf. page 109).

the past the slogan of child care used to be: Rest, Regularity and Cleanliness, reflecting an attitude which particularly had the protection of the child in mind. Strengthening the social position of young people was hardly or not at all discussed. This attitude was perhaps satisfactory in a period in which the course of a child's life was mainly determined by religion, tradition and birth, and so seemed a more or less natural constant. Nowadays, not only have the individual options for the young increased considerably (du Bois-Reymond, 1992), but we have also become aware of the relation between their development possibilities and the chances given to them by society. For this reason a new slogan was proposed, the three Rs, Rights, Room and Respect for the young (de Winter, 1990, page 27). 'The young deserve the future' not only because they are valuable capital becoming scarce due to the de-greening of society and because society invests a lot in their training and care. Quite apart from that young people have a Right to personal integrity, a Right to good facilities and also a Right to a future. They need material and emotional Room to grow up, to play, but also need to be able to actually explore society, otherwise than through abstract information. And they deserve Respect and appreciation by adults so as to come to feel that their existence constitutes a meaningful element of culture. Participation by children and young people is to be considered an essential way of realizing these three principles. There is however one more reason to plead for participation. There are namely valid arguments for the assumption that the lack of opportunities for participation has a negative influence on the psychosocial well-being of young people. Whereas conversely the promotion of active commitment appears to influence the development of young people in a positive sense. For this reason the stimulation of participation may be considered a preventive or even curative intervention which may prevent or counteract problems of young people. Granted, it is a little peculiar to legitimize a fundamental and just ideal for education that should be pursued for all young people, on the basis of preventive or therapeutic value. At the same time however, this shows the basic value of such an ideal. The need for active social commitment is obviously so essential, that its frustration may considerably restrict the developmental possibilities of young people and may even cause various problems in psychosocial well being. In the light of this we may consider participation to be a basic need, and therefore a *basic right with a beneficial effect.*

Participation by children and young people is not an entirely new idea. Extensive experiments, sometimes under somewhat different labels, have been going on in practice in the fields of youth welfare work, community work, and education. Notions of this kind are to be found in disciplines such as youth sociology, educational theory and developmental psychology. Participation by young people, as a means and aim of social education, could be taken to be *old wine in new bottles.* There is much to be learnt, however, from this old wine. This is why most chapters of this book start with an excursion into the past. The objective is not so much to write full biographies of fields of practice or science, but especially to show in what circumstances such ideas and experiments in various domains could take root or could die a gentle or violent death. This historicizing approach may moreover provide an insight into the question why participation and social commitment are now such scant themes in youth policy, youth work and in youth and educational studies.

One of the conceivable objections that could be raised against the promotion of participation is the fact that, in the past, young people were frequently invited or even forced to participate in social activities that served not so much their own development, but ideological targets of adults. In this connection movements such as the Hitlerjugend and the youth movements of the communist parties in the former Eastern bloc are usually referred to. But according to some theoreticians the voluntary way in which young people in democratic societies are employed in realizing various political and ideological targets can also be interpreted as a *subtle, modern strategy of fitting them in.* For this reason we shall try to work out carefully what the various objects and effects of participation are or were, and especially, with what ideal for the future has this notion been connected in the course of time. This is one of the reasons for relating participation to the concept of citizenship, for some people a perhaps somewhat stale concept. It is exactly the historically changing meanings of this term which clearly indicate what, in the various periods, was expected and demanded from young people as future citizens. Following naturally from this, one may wonder what the material basis is for a social ideal of education which considers young persons to be fellow citizens. In other words: how realistic is it to demand of young people that they show civic responsibility and behaviour, when for many of them there are only uncertain perspectives. Phenomena such as high unemployment among young people and marginalization of large groups of young people do not work as stimuli in this context. For this reason the promotion of the participation by children and young people cannot be regarded as a universal remedy for all social problems that manifest themselves around this category of fellow citizens. We make no pretence to this in this book. Our line of approach is particularly that of social education: an essential, but not in itself sufficient condition for juvenile citizenship. Another conceivable objection is that the ideas presented here have long become widely accepted. Has the plea to see children as fellow citizens not long been overtaken by the reality of the 'negotiating household' in which young people have their own views on just about everything? And are their rights not sufficiently safeguarded now that the UN Convention on the Rights of Children has recently been accepted? To answer such questions we look at concrete educational practice in the family, the neighbourhood, the school and youth social work. There is hardly any reliable quantitative research into the actual spread of participation by children in these domains. This can be simply explained by the fact that it has so far not been a very popular subject of research. For that reason we often have to use indirect sources, such as research done with other objectives, policy memoranda and practical experience. In a sense this study is a preliminary exploration of the terrain, indeed endeavouring to make points of view and findings acceptable, but in which not every statement or conclusion can be underpinned empirically.

The book is structured as follows. In the first part the theoretical framework of participation by children and young people is reviewed. In Chapter 1 we discuss the phenomenon that young people are viewed mainly as a problem. This serves as a counterpoint to the development of a participation perspective (Chapter 2), in which the position and opportunities of children are looked at on the basis of modern ideas on citizenship and education for citizenship. In Chapter 3 we successively discuss the ways in which pedagogy and developmental psychology have been, are, and could be looking at this phenomenon. In part two we discuss three fields of practice in which participation is of great importance, namely local youth policy (Chapter 4), education (Chapter 5) and professional youth care (Chapter 6). Chapter 7 contains the concluding observations, in which the critical considerations mentioned earlier are looked at again.

References

Bois-Reymond M du (1992) *Jongeren op weg naar volwassenheid*. Groningen: Wolters-Noordhoff.

Hazekamp JL, J van der Gauw & J Nuijens (1993) *Jongeren doen mee aan beleid. Verslag van een onderzoek naar politieke participatie van jongeren op lokaal niveau*. 's-Gravenhage: VNG.

Ministerie van Welzijn, Volksgezondheid en Cultuur (1991) *Samenwerken langs nieuwe wegen*. 's-Gravenhage: WVC.

Winter M de (1990) *De kwaliteit van het kinderlijk bestaan*. Oratie Universiteit Utrecht. Bunnik: Landelijke Vereniging voor Thuiszorg.

Part One

The young: a generation full of problems

Introduction

In 1992 two government agencies in the Netherlands, the Socio-Cultural Planning Agency (Sociaal en Cultureel Planbureau SCP) and the Scientific Advisory Board on Government Policy (Wetenschappelijke Raad voor het Regeringsbeleid WRR) each published a study on the situation of the young in the Netherlands. The two reports differ considerably in tone, but the factual findings are roughly the same: the greater part, some 80%, of young people are doing well in various respects, but some 20% have considerable problems (ter Bogt & van Praag, 1992; Diekstra, 1992). There is, however, a striking contrast between the conclusions drawn from each study: whereas the Socio-Cultural Planning Agency concludes that young people are generally doing well, an image of woe prevails in the WRR report. There has been much speculation and discussion on the background to this considerable difference in interpretation (cf. van Praag, 1993; Diekstra, 1993; Meeus, 1993). Here, however, the discrepancy as such is more important than the reasons as it shows that concepts about young people may be evoked more or less independently of the true situation. If this is the case to such an extent with research workers, we should have few illusions about the factual basis of images current among social workers, policy makers, politicians and the general public. A strong preoccupation with problems characterizes the present socio-political climate with regard to today's young people. Although the media and commerce do their best with catchy slogans to define this phase of life as 'enjoying freedom, adventure, a beautiful body and a life without cares ' (Dieleman & Perreijn, 1993, page 16), the same media almost daily give us cause for alarm with their items on the disinterest and lack of standards, on vandalism, materialism, dropping out of school and criminality among 'the young'.

'*Young people cause problems, young people have problems*'; a statement made by the Netherlands Government in a recent policy document (Ministry of Welfare, Public Health and Cultural Affairs WVC, 1993). Research workers in this field also sounded the alarm. Based on a number of literature studies[2] Meeus (1993) concludes that post-war

---

[2]cf. Abma (1986) among others.

research has been strongly oriented towards *ad hoc* handling of problems, towards problem youngsters and sub-sectors of the world of the young. On the basis of research into problem youngsters the whole generation is thus declared a problem category. Of course all this is not to imply that no problems exist, or that they should be played down. There is ample reason for society to be concerned about some young people. About one fifth contending with serious problems is no small matter[3]. Moreover the rise in this percentage between 1970 and 1990 is a reason for action. The generalization of these problems, in the public's conception of large groups of children and young people, requires critical analysis, however. One-sided, disproportionate attention given to the negative aspects of youth may be considered a threat to the social and educational climate in which they grow up. After all, looking at young people through problem-tinted spectacles impedes one's view of their positive qualities and potential. This is why it is important to discover the sources of the culture of problems that has developed around children and young people. In this chapter we ask ourselves why in the course of history adults have so strongly stressed the difficulties that young people have, and cause. To what extent does an actual occurrence of problems play a part? Taking three types of children who serve as models for the thinking about young people by today's society, we shall examine how this problematization works nowadays.

Historical backgrounds to the youth problem

History of the family and upbringing

During the past decades heated debates have been held on the question as to how the treatment of young people by adults has developed in history. Some historians say that adult compassion towards the young has grown in the course of centuries, others conclude that on the contrary 'loving' children is more a kind of constant factor in human evolution. We shall not enter into this historians' debate in detail. We shall just listen to a few authoritative voices to indicate the direction into which the association of grown-ups and young people has evolved. Lloyd DeMause (1974) used an extensive study of source material to develop a division into historical phases of parental behaviour towards children. According to him, up to the beginning of the Middle Ages parents did not flinch from killing their children if

---

[3]The Netherlands Council for Youth Policy (Raad voor het Jeugdbeleid) in its report 'Aanval op Uitval' (Fighting dropping-out) (1994) mentions between 10 and 15 per cent of young people having serious or multiple problems. Such differences arise because identical definitions of 'problems' are by no means always used.

circumstances demanded; until the thirteenth century it was not unusual to get rid of them in various ways (giving away, abandonment). From that period onwards however, parental empathy grows: until 1600, it is true, an ambivalent attitude prevails (interest and subjection), but gradually this attitude changes into educational practices in which the feelings of and for the child play an ever greater part. According to DeMause the eighteenth century is characterized by a recognition of the typical character of the child as one who deserves special interest and attention, but whose urges must be checked and obedience enforced. In the following century 'control' is gradually replaced by 'socialization'; education takes on the character of guidance to adulthood, the child has to learn to meet the demands the world makes on it. The last phase, according to DeMause, starts after the First World War. Parents increasingly address the child's needs and thus become its helper and servant.

Although DeMause's work has frequently been criticized, among other things because of his one-sided psychological interpretations[4], many other authors in general share his ideas on the direction of historical shifts. Since the seventeenth and eighteenth centuries the attitude towards children seems to have been subject to significant changes. One of the most radical points of view is held by Philippe Ariès, who more or less denies the existence of a separate juvenile world before the beginning of modern times (Ariès, 1987). In his view there was hardly any question of upbringing in the Middle Ages, because children from about the age of seven were incorporated in the adult world without a clear transitional phase. He contrasts this period with the Hellenic era, in which there was a clear demarcation between the worlds of adults and children, marked by initiation rites, training and education. According to Ariès the period of upbringing, and with it the modern child, finally came into being by the end of the seventeenth century. Under the influence of the clergy parents were persuaded that they themselves were responsible for the spiritual and physical welfare of their children. Parental care led to the development of a new type of affective relations ('loving care') between parents and children; parents had the moral duty to prepare children, girls as well as boys, for adult life. Children were obliged to attend school, under a strict regime, and shut off from the outside world[5].

---

[4]For a critical view see among others Spiecker & Groenendijk (1980) and Roos & Boswinkel (1981).

[5]The views held by Ariès have also raised heated argument among family historians. Peeters (1975), who on the basis of his own research concludes that at the beginning of the modern era (1500–1650) there was a recognition already of the typical character of children and young people, blames the lack of consensus in this matter mainly on careless use of historical sources. The differences in views and interpretation anyway relate more specifically to the historical position of younger children; views on the position of young people are more

Historian Linda Pollock (1983) however believes that parents' love of their children is not such a modern phenomenon. From her study, covering the period from 1500–1900, she draws the conclusion that strong ties between parents and children have to be considered a historical continuity. Noordman & van Setten (1989) put this division into perspective by pointing out the changes in the conditions that have shaped the interaction between parents and children through the centuries: 'the question is not whether parents in the past did or did not love their children, the question is rather whether in the past they always commanded sufficient insight, knowledge and material possibilities to shape the emotional ties with their children in the modern way' (page 153). The fact that in the eighteenth and nineteenth centuries very many children were abandoned, cannot in their view simply be interpreted as lack of parental love, but should be seen as the inevitable consequence of extreme poverty among large parts of the population. The same applies to the employment of young children in the production process or in households. The fact that children often had to do heavy work and put in long hours from the age of six, had to do with bitter economic necessity rather than with parental indifference. Even well into the twentieth century many poor families could hardly afford the luxury of a protective youthland. For the time being this was a privilege of the well-to-do, in whose circles a clear tendency has indeed been observed, since the seventeenth and eighteenth centuries, to spend more time and attention on care and education. The Enlightenment ideal of the practically unlimited possibilities to educate children (see Chapter 4) was an important source of inspiration. This intensification of education could only take shape within the less well-off part of the population when the elementary conditions of life also improved somewhat, for instance in the form of better housing. The changes in the relations between children and parents are therefore strongly associated with the conditions in which people live, and large differences in the rate of development are apparent in different social environments. Nevertheless it can be argued that in the course of centuries education has increasingly turned into a special activity. On the one hand parents were held more strictly responsible for upbringing, on the other hand they themselves began to feel that they had such a responsibility.

Civilization and professionalization

Elias (1982) sees these changes in the relationship between parents and children against the background of a wider process of civilization. In the

---

unanimous according to Peeters. With regard to this group the eighteenth century is generally considered to be the period in which youth as a category comes into being, or at least changes character drastically. For this debate see also: Röling (1982) and Noordman & van Setten (1989).

course of European history, affected by the formation of nation-states, the monopolization of violence by the state, economic differentiation and changes in power and class relations, people have become increasingly interdependent. Such social changes, accompanied by changes in the nature of human relationships, have also had a far-reaching influence on the development of the personality structure of successive generations. This psychic and relational process of civilization is particularly characterized by the increasing control of human passions; people learn to rein in spontaneous passions and to relate their own actions to the consequences for others. This transformation, which in fact also takes place within individual development, moves from high to low and from without to within. Rules and standards first come into being in elitist circles, are then imposed on and adopted by lower strata, and are gradually internalized. This process has far-reaching consequences, especially for the relations between parents and children. Since the regulation of emotions and behaviour has become a critical sign of individual civilization and at the same time a condition for achieving social status, family education is becoming more and more important. Self-control as a social standard requires careful disciplining of children, because their misbehaviour poses a threat to the cultural level and prestige that parents are trying to acquire. At the same time that education was being intensified, the physical gap between parents and children was increasing. If they were to civilize the young, they had to shield them from everything that could threaten their childish innocence, such as sexuality. Moreover teachers increasingly took over socializing tasks from the family. In fact school offered to prepare children for adulthood by keeping them at a distance from harsh reality for a longer time.

de Swaan (1989) also relates the evolution of human relationships to larger processes of social change. The development of social amenities such as education, health services and social security are at the core of his analysis. He views the creation of *public services* and the resulting *professional regimes* as the outcome of the social struggle that took place between the various elitist groups (the Establishment). These groups endeavoured to avert the threat posed by the poor, and at the same time to exploit the possibilities of cheap and disciplined labour. The spread of primary education, for instance, was accompanied by fierce conflicts between municipal elites and the burgeoning state machinery on the one hand, and the landed gentry and the clergy on the other. It was not so much the educational ideas that were at stake, but the possibilities education afforded to control and regulate the poor. Conservative circles have always been extremely afraid of any subversive effect general education could have on the common people. In contrast, their opponents stressed the opportunities for improvement: education for the general population could eliminate the 'bias, stubbornness and rebelliousness of the peasants and put an end to idleness and vice in the young, while a better understanding of the moral basis of society could even prevent a rising of the masses' (ibid., page 66).

The organization of collective social amenities has been accompanied, particularly in the present century, by the rise of professional elites that came to occupy a mediatory position between state and population. For instance, medical and educational regimes were gradually established, and to a considerable extent began to structure the needs, behaviour and problems of the population. More and more realms of life fell under the direct control of experts. Education is a case in point because it did not only lay a heavy claim on young people's time, but at the same time thrust numerous arrangements and standards upon the family. Personal lives were also greatly influenced by the indirect effects of these professional regimes. People learned to translate their experiences and problems within the framework of notions handed out to them by experts. While this 'proto-professionalization' facilitated client access to professionals, it also enabled professionals to enlarge their domains. Gradually lay people appropriated the abstract language of the experts, so that these regimes were not experienced as actual coercion. By now this proto-professionalization has become a kind of cultural hallmark. Parents have learned to regard their children as potential carriers of disturbance or problems; they 'know' how great their own influence is on the origin and prevention of such problems (de Winter, 1986). And children also learn that they have an active share in the relational problems arising between them and their parents. For instance, in the subject 'care', as introduced in the new curriculum for the lower forms of secondary schools, the course of the pupil's development and the family conflicts that may be part of it are addressed at some length.

Post-structuralist theoreticians like Foucault (1975) and Donzelot (1979) point out the regulating and productive effect emanating from these professional regimes. Their strength is not so much in the prescribing of new educational or therapeutic methods, but in the creation of an ostensibly neutral argument that gave problems a psychological meaning. People who do not observe generally accepted standards are no longer excluded; they are first problematized and subsequently fitted in and integrated into society, albeit by persuasion and preferably of their own free will. This 'psycomplex' provided both a language and a practice that enabled intervention in families without this being experienced as coercion. Thus authorities could steer family life in the right direction, experts could extend their domain, and mothers in particular rose in esteem because their responsibility for raising children was increasingly appreciated. The sociologist Ingrid van Lieshout criticizes this view, notably because of the one-sided influence it ascribes to experts. In this context she prefers to speak of the advent of a 'problem culture', in which experts as well as laity are continuously oriented towards all potential problems in all conceivable realms of life. She stresses potential problems since cultural susceptibilities address not only tangible difficulties, but especially 'problems that may arise in the future, problems experienced by others and/or problems that occurred in the past' (van Lieshout, 1993).

Greater empathy of parents with children, civilization, proto-professionalization and a gradual postponement of adulthood: this is the picture sketched so far of the historical changes that have occurred with regard to young people. These developments may be considered significant conditions for the process of the problematization of young people as put forward at the beginning of this chapter. Under the influence of such changes, more and more intensive attention has been paid to children and young people; it is as if they are permanently under a magnifying glass. According to Schnabel, they have become 'an increasingly precious cultural heritage'. Notably from the nineteenth century onwards, their 'self-evident presence in a world of adults and children has made way for the attendance, meticulously directed, of selected third parties around them: in the upbringing of children and the pattern of their world, the only self-evident thing is that nothing is self-evident any more. Everything is regulated by scientifically legitimate ideas on what, at what point in time, to what extent and offered by whom is in fact "good" for the child's development'. This psychological and social upgrading of the child first took place in the upper middle class. For the proletariat of the nineteenth century, the value of their children at first only decreased. Since the industrialization and the migration to the towns children had been less and less of an insurance for old age. The rise in the number of children per family, resulting from a drastic reduction in infant mortality, caused growing poverty. However, the rise in prosperity, culminating in the twentieth century welfare state, established the ideal of youth having a right to protection and development as a social standard for all layers of the population (Schnabel, 1992). This turned the modern child into a highly prized 'possession', but at the same time into the cause of more and more concern and anxiety. After all, the higher the social ideals and requirements, the stronger the pressure to put them into practice[6].

To gain a better understanding of the specific mechanism of problematization we are going to introduce three contemporary children, each representing an important style of modern thinking on youth problems. We review in turn the 'predictable child', the 'social renewal child', and the 'moral rearmament child'.

---

[6]The processes of social change described here are naturally accompanied by developments in educational ideas and practice. These are treated extensively in Chapter 3 on child-raising and development and in Chapter 5 on education.

The predictable child

Developments in health care and medical technology, as well as the increased knowledge and influence of psychology and educational science, have created greater opportunities for the early detection of problems in children's development, sometimes even prenatally. Many parents seem pleased with these triumphs of modern capabilities, believing that now unnecessarily serious consequences of problems can be avoided. The time is long past that children were only discovered to have hearing impairments at primary school, since hearing is now systematically tested in the first year of life, at the well-baby clinic. It is now equally feasible to assess the development of speech and language at an early stage, so that interventions can take place much earlier than they used to be. To give better shape and substance to early detection of developmental disorders, so-called VTO-teams (VTO = early detection of developmental problems) were formed in the Netherlands in the seventies and eighties. The main aim of their multidisciplinary cooperation was to shorten the route parents often have to travel through the social services when they suspect something is not right with their child.

New technology and improved procedures within social services have made children's development more predictable (cf. de Winter, 1986). This is an unmistakable gain, but there is a price to pay. The practice of early detection of problems and disorders represents a major change in our culture. The influence of experts and their disciplines on development is steadily increasing. Almost daily new methods are presented for screening, prenatal examination and pedagogic recognition of signals. Parents adopt the language and notions of professionals: 'doctor, my son still does not use two-word sentences', or: 'do you think Bianca suffers under her acquired helplessness?' To improve prospects for early detection it was thought important to raise the sensitivity to signals of all those who had to do with children. Firstly parents, but also kindergarten teachers, teachers, baby clinic doctors and district nurses should become parts of a warning network. For this purpose each of these categories had to be trained in aspects of normal and abnormal development. Although the discussion on early detection has by now passed its peak it has left clear traces in today's thinking on children. The 'predictable child' may be considered a symbol of a social attitude, in which a possible defect or disorder largely determines the actions of professionals and parents towards their children. The pursuit, in itself laudable, of early detection has had the side-effect that children's potential problems have increasingly influenced the practice of upbringing (ibid.).

The social renewal child

Since the end of the eighties youth policy has gradually become interested in a new type of child, who again could be considered the symbol of the child image in our society. This child came into being during the process of social renewal, a Dutch policy programme – by now faded – of the Christian Democrat/Social Democrat administration (1989–1994) aimed at halting the marginalization of underprivileged groups of the population. The social renewal child is included in these high-risk groups. It is a member of an ethnic minority, or perhaps lives in one of the areas of multiple deprivation in the big cities. Clearly it cannot just be found anywhere, for welfare work has developed a new procedure to meet it: the so-called catchment place method. The locations are defined as 'low threshold facilities where many children are to be found, for example the baby clinic, day care, primary school or community centre'. There also seems quite a lot the matter with this child. It belongs to at-risk groups for a whole range of personal and social problems, such as abuse, language deficiency, poor school performance, truancy, dropping out of school, family problems, criminality and in later life, unemployment. It grows up in families characterized by an accumulation of stress, psychic and social problems, financial problems, addiction, violence, poor housing, discrimination and so forth. The social renewal child has a growing number of professional interventions at its disposal. Many sectors are specifically active in prevention and social work: youth health care, child day care, social services for children, schools and welfare agencies. For the social renewal child, preventive activities are mainly concentrated at the neighbourhood level. Signals from children about whom concern is felt are regularly discussed within the 'interdisciplinary neighbourhood networks for social youth work' formed in many places. The social workers and educators directly concerned cooperate in deciding how the child and the family can best be supported. Parents receive individually aimed educational support, they are coached with video home training or low-key educational counselling. In the pre-school period parents may be coached in the cognitive development of their children with the aid of compensation programmes. The aim of this type of counselling is to prevent the child already being irreparably disadvantaged on entering primary school.

Such developments have clearly shifted the emphasis in youth policy. The general orientation towards developmental disorders that could concern all children has become an orientation towards a specific problem group: the underprivileged children in society. There appear to be various reasons and arguments for this. First there is an *economic* motive: it would seem more efficient to target preventive activities at groups that will give rise to the highest cost in later stages of social work, education and health care.

Secondly social *solidarity* plays a part in this policy: within the framework of social renewal, politicians want to address the groups that have the fewest social opportunities. Thirdly it is partly prompted by social *angst*: such prevention concerns not only children in danger, but also dangerous children or at least children society expects to be dangerous. Finally *professional* motives play a part: for some professional groups, such as educationalists and psychologists, the social renewal child provides access to a group of clients previously almost closed to them, while other groups, that had already long been concerned with these categories of children, acquire new tasks.

As a concept the social renewal child poses a few essential problems. First of all the term 'at-risk group', so characteristic of this child, is debatable in both a scientific and a social sense. To describe such a group accurately one must have sufficient knowledge and understanding of the causes of the problem which could constitute a risk. If such knowledge is incomplete, explanatory factors are often attributed to more or less chance characteristics. This was, for instance, the case with autism, the cause of which was long thought to have lain in the unemotional reactions of the mother. So-called cold mothers were thus designated as being at-risk for having autistic children. Many years and large numbers of wrongly stigmatized mothers later, it was concluded that cause and effect had been confused. The same difficulty now presents itself with regard to the social renewal child as the representative of an at-risk group. In the case of this child very complex, multiple problems are concerned, and it is not possible to indicate a simple cause. If this is nevertheless done, for instance by just designating 'member of an ethnic minority' as a risk characteristic, the effect will be stigmatizing and discriminatory. Whether an ethnic child or parent is doing well or badly, they will be considered part of a group that has something wrong with it. Thus they will become the target of interventions because of their origin.

A second problem for the social renewal child lies in the individualizing character of the intervention strategies that have been worked out for it. Children's health and well-being depend on a complexity of factors to be sought within the individual, but also in the social context. The social renewal child is particularly characterized by a build-up of social problems that present themselves in neighbourhoods with numerous deprivation cases. The majority of the interventions within the framework of social renewal youth policy however target individual children and parents. This produces the impression that it is they themselves that are at the core of the problem, perhaps because of poor educational abilities (cf. de Winter, 1992).

The moral rearmament child

While the social renewal child is still alive and kicking (witness the numerous educational support and pre-school stimulation projects now being carried out everywhere in the Western World) it has meanwhile got a major competitor. The combating of deprivation as a social priority seems to have been supplanted by the combating of its supposed dangers: delinquency, vandalism, vagrancy, fraud, misuse of social services and so on. In this context a social and political atmosphere ensues in which the decline of public morality is blamed for all kinds of social ills. With regard to young people an image emerges of the blurring of standards and lack of responsibility, blamed partly on themselves, partly on their educators. The problem of rising juvenile delinquency is said to be mainly due to inadequate 'moral' education at home and in schools. This proposition, hard to prove in itself, served as a guideline for numerous political speeches and propositions in the early nineties: exhortations to parents to pay more attention to standards and values, lessons in moral reasoning at school, strengthening of the educational task of schools, boot camp for seriously derailed youngsters, etc. In short: young people, via parents, school and the law, should be morally rearmed[7]. Because at this same time all sorts of provisions for young persons (social benefits, study grants) were cut, some called this an attack on, or even a 'war against the young' (Heemskerk, 1993; Helder, 1993).

Such propositions flourish in a social climate in which so-called excesses of the welfare state are a welcome subject of discussion. Young people, just like other categories among the public, are said to have been too pampered, and to have undermined the foundations of the welfare state by their calculating, irresponsible behaviour. That educators in particular will be apportioned the blame in such a discussion, is self-evident. The problems are, after all, caused by the state having taken too many tasks and responsibilities away from the ordinary citizen. The allegation that the decline of values and standards is the cause of juvenile delinquency or of its increase, is contested by many. Junger-Tas, who for that matter qualifies this rise as such[8], emphasizes on the basis of various research that there is

---

[7]This term is used because of the parallel with the ideas of the movement of that name founded by the Reverend Buchman in Oxford in 1921. This Christian philanthropic movement advocated the saving of the world order through moral renewal of personal life; the values considered suitable were then formulated in more absolute terms than is now usually the case, however.

[8]cf. also van der Laan (1993), who on the basis of recent research data rejects the frequently stated conclusion that juvenile delinquency is strongly on the rise and is becoming more and more serious as a whole.

hardly any question of such a decline. It is true that secularization and individualization make morals less and less unequivocal, but on the other hand behaviour that used to be tolerated, such as violence within the family, is rejected more and more strongly. She lists as main causes for the rise in juvenile delinquency: (1) the increased percentage of young people since the Second World War, (2) the increased prosperity and the attendant growth of opportunities to commit offences, and (3) decreased control and supervision of young people. In her opinion it is not so much a question of deviating morals, as of poor enforcement (Junger-Tas, 1993). The cultural sociologist Zijderveld (1992) has a similar point of view, when he maintains that in society actions are increasingly detached from their consequences. Standards and values (with young people and educators) are not, according to him, absent as such, but 'are free-floating: abstract and noncommittal'. He made this statement at a meeting convened by the Netherlands Ministry of Justice on the subject of socially prescriptive education. Practically all those present shared the opinion that social supervision of young persons should be strengthened. Opinions differed greatly, however, on the way in which this should be done, notably on what the respective roles of the authorities, the educational system and the family should be (Ministry of Justice, 1992). Whether young people ought to receive better moral education in the home and at school, or whether social supervision of them ought to be intensified, it is clear that the attitudes and behaviour of the young increasingly evoke apprehensive concern in adults. In so far as social factors play any part in the debate, they practically always concern criticism of too much permissiveness and indulgence, or in this case failing social control. The criminologists Witte and Yesilgöz (1992) sharply criticize the one-sided character of this 'social control theory' which they say dominates the policies and research concerning juvenile delinquency; in this way not only does the influence of socio-economic conditions (financial problems, poor housing conditions, etc.) disappear from sight, but whole groups of the population, especially ethnic minorities, are criminalized and marginalized. It is, after all, their background situation which is held responsible for a considerable part of juvenile delinquency.

Education without standards and values is by definition impossible, both at home and at school. The plea for moral rearmament of young people should therefore be interpreted as criticism of the nature and substance of current educational morals, not so much of a lack of them. Zijderveld denounces this as 'morals of the risk of being caught', in which behaviour is not so much steered by a collective sense of good and evil, but by a functional and rationalistic profit and loss account drawn up by each individual in each situation (Zijderveld, 1992). Based on this train of thought, society has to compel young people and educators, or at least earnestly stimulate them, to reverse the decline. Here, however, closing the gap between behaviour and consequences creates a new gap; the gap between morals and the actual circumstances under which people live, grow up and educate. The moral rearmament child should therefore be considered the product of a social strategy that aims to lay the responsibility for social problems at the door of the problem groups themselves. It is not so much a question of disadvantages but of wilful default[9].

Youth as a three-dimensional problem

These three ways of thinking about young people each present their own picture of 'youth as a problem'. In these various pictures different analyses can be identified of the way in which the causes, consequences and possible solutions of youth problems are viewed. From a theoretical point of view these various analyses could be arranged along the lines of so-called aggregation levels, that is to say that explanatory factors are differentiated at micro-, meso-, and macro- levels (cf. among others Bronfenbrenner, 1979; see page 59). We are not concerned here only with explanations of the problematic behaviour itself, but with an analysis of the way in which in various types of youth policy the problematization process is given shape. Therefore we have selected a line of approach based on some major mechanisms which are active in the social problematization process. These are generalization, individualization and effect assignment.

Generalization

Early detection of development disorders, as well as projects within the framework of social renewal youth policy and initiatives around the theme of socially prescriptive education, may be conceived as preventive activities. Although the aims as well as the means chosen diverge widely, they share the characteristic that in the first instance they target a (more or less carefully) defined problem area and the connected group. In the case of early detection the targets are the (threatening) development disorders in children between birth and the age of seven. For the educational support and pre-school stimulation (social renewal youth policy) projects, psychosocial problems and arrears in cognitive development are concerned, notably in young children (up to 6 years) in socially deprived circumstances. The discussions and propositions with regard to socially prescriptive education in general target young people of all ages who already demonstrate delinquent behaviour or are at risk to do so. The emphasis is unmistakably on marginal groups, notably ethnic young people.

---

[9]In Chapter 5 we treat the question of values and standards in education in greater detail.

Prevention generally entails informing, examining, screening or checking a much larger group than the number of persons who actually have the targeted problem. This means that a problem group is necessarily generalized to a potential problem group. In the same way, to decrease mortality from cardiac and vascular disorders, the entire population is informed about the risks of high fat consumption and smoking. And, in order to detect as many cases of breast cancer as possible at an early stage, all women between 55 and 70 are regularly called up for screening – and here an at-risk group is indeed concerned. We have already pointed out the scientific problems involved in defining such groups. The more ambiguous the targets[10] of prevention are, and the less is known about the origin and course of the problem, the more difficult it is to define the at-risk groups. Should the definition be made on an unsound basis, it will inevitably lead to false stigmatization.

The prevention of development disorders, and of problems of deprivation and deviant behaviour also has to do with such a generalization. In the case of early detection the whole of the child population from birth to the age of seven became a prevention target. The new element in this approach, of course, was that potential disorders were emphatically brought to the attention of everybody who either privately or professionally had to do with parents and children. Information campaigns were held in which the signalling task of adults was explicitly pointed out. People learned to look at all children as potential problem carriers (cf. de Winter, 1986). Social renewal youth policy entails a different generalization. In order to find those families where educational problems, perhaps in the form of insufficient cognitive stimulation, arise at an early stage, all parents with young children from so-called disadvantaged groups or neighbourhoods constituted the target group for preventive support. Defining such a rough at-risk group, together with the individual preventive approach selected, led to the problematization of all young people in a disadvantaged situation. In this way it is not the situation itself, but the children and their parents, who become subjects of preventive policies.

'Moral rearmament' is attended by a comparable generalization. Here too a fairly restricted group of young people is the real target group, but the intended remedy is declared applicable to a much wider category. For the time being the group of young people (families) targeted is recruited from among 'the' disadvantaged groups, notably ethnic minorities. But according to many who take part in this broad social discussion, the call for reinforcement of standards and values in fact concerns everybody. The plea for the pedagogic task of the education system points in this direction.

---

[10]'Targets' in health care, and notably in the World Health Organization denote 'aims of prevention'.

To sum up: generalization, i.e. the (potential) attribution of the characteristics of a limited group to a much larger population, is an inherent part of a preventive strategy based on at-risk groups. Whether or not this larger population possesses the characteristics looked for, is immaterial in so far as establishing an image is concerned. As witnessed by public opinion on ethnic young people, stigmatization proves to have an effect. In this sense generalization has to be considered a major dimension of the problematization of young people.

Individualization

Through generalization the group of young people suspected of certain problems is growing. But to what extent is the cause of their problems also to be found in them or within their families? The answer to this question clearly contributes to the extent to which youth can be considered a problem. It is difficult of course, to make any general pronouncements here, since the pattern of causal factors is different for each specific problem field. Scientists however have long been in agreement on the principle that behaviour and development are the effects of dynamic interaction between the individual and his surroundings (cf. Sameroff, 1975). With respect to health and welfare there is a more or less similar consensus. The so-called ecological health model used by the World Health Organization in their programme *Health for All by the Year 2000* lists five determinants for health and well-being. They are physical factors, personal behaviour, social environment, physical environment and the quality of the system of care (Lalonde, 1974).

Comparing the types of youth policy described above with scientific opinion, we are struck by the one-sidedness of the interpretation of problems around young people. The emphasis is practically always on the micro level of individual behaviour, individual development and family relationships. Often environmental factors, such as socio-economic status, discrimination or housing are mentioned, but usually as independent variables. That is to say, they do not constitute explicit targets for intervention. This process, in which complex causal relations are reduced to intra- or inter-personal factors, is sometimes called individualization[11]. It has a certain logic, because influencing the relevant environmental factor is a very difficult matter and is not always supported by a political majority. An example: it is well-known that young people from an ethnic minority, even if they have completed schooling, have a considerably inferior labour

---

[11]The term is not here used in the meaning of a social development in which individuals are and/or want to be increasingly more self-sufficient.

market perspective to that of indigenous youngsters. Alleviating this situation would involve active intervention in the labour market. In many countries it has proved fairly difficult to do this, even though such a lack of perspective is indicated as a source of crime and marginalization. On the other hand, there is broad support for a strategy to try and equip individual children from ethnic minorities better for a successful school career: the pre-school stimulation programme. Without questioning its usefulness this is clearly an individualizing approach. This means that the individualization process burdens young people and their families with a personal responsibility for problems which can only partly be justified in the light of present scientific insight. People who get the idea that society holds them individually responsible for things they themselves can barely influence, inevitably feel frustration, which may be turned inwards or outwards. This explains the anger, impotence, indifference or apathy which gradually takes control of many marginalized young people. In a socio-political sense the process of individualization constitutes a justification of policy that is unfriendly towards the young. If deviation from standards by young people is made out to be mainly a behavioural or educational problem, politics have no option but repressive measures. It is then easy to invoke the thesis that 'neither employment policies nor training programmes can cope with character disorders or parental failure' (Halsema & Coppes, 1993, page 11).

To sum up: individualization is a process which locates the causes of problematic behaviour mainly at intra- or inter-personal level. For young people and parents this results in an apportioning of responsibility or blame which is only partially justified. In this sense the process has a stigmatizing effect (just as in the case of generalization), and contributes in no small measure to the creation of a problem image of young people.

Effect assignment

The question as to whom the burden of problems concerning the young should be assigned is the last dimension of problematization to be discussed here. After all, it is not immaterial to the establishment of an image whether the effects of disorders, disadvantages or deviant behaviour are laid at the door of the individual child (or family), or at that of the general public. The word 'effects' does not so much refer to financial and factual consequences of these problems, but rather to the effects that people feel (the subjective perception). In this context we should of course take into consideration that the types of problems under discussion in the various categories of youth policies are not absolutely identical. It is however possible to indicate a common denominator. Research into the case-load of the Dutch Early Detection teams has shown that the disorders reported are chiefly behavioural problems and problems (delays) in cognitive development

(Bosga, 1993). These are the exact areas of attention targeted by the projects 'educational support to measure' and 'pre-school stimulation programme', while socially prescriptive education is also targeted at behavioural problems. When considering the three methods described above, we see a clear shift in the assignment of effects. The *predictable child* was itself, together with its parents, clearly the victim. It was generally seen as a child that had to be approached with great compassion. Publications on early detection in the sixties, seventies and eighties were generally characterized by a large measure of understanding of, and commitment to, the parents facing problems and uncertainties. The essential message was: a developmental disorder is a fate that hits a parent through no fault of his or her own, and therefore she or he has a right to the best possible support. In the case of the *social renewal child* there is mixed assignment of effects. In the memorandum 'Educational Support to Measure' the target group is denoted as vulnerable young people: they are children who suffer from a cumulation of threatening circumstances of a personal and social nature. Early intervention is deemed necessary, because 'otherwise they will get into a downward spiral, leading from bad to worse'. (In this context, 'worse' indicated those 'untreatable' young persons who are not only victims themselves, but could also constitute a social risk.) (Ministry of Welfare, Public Health and Cultural Affairs WVC, 1992). The *moral rearmament child* finally has been created solely because of its dangers for society. However, in all the discussions on socially prescriptive education, we have been unable to find references to any possible harmful effects that moral decline could have on young people themselves.

To sum up: the various styles of youth policy we have considered mainly target the same types of youth problems, but diverge sharply in situating the effects of these problems. Early detection clearly places the problem with parent and child, social renewal youth policy introduces a mixture of personal and social effects, while socially prescriptive education is exclusively aimed at combatting social risks.

Conclusions

The problematization of young people, as we argued, may partly be understood from a number of global socio-cultural processes of change such as the intensified interest in young people, in civilization and (proto)professionalization. In this sense it may be considered to fit in with the modernization of western societies. One aspect that plays a part in this is an increasing, though implicit social control of young people, not so much by the state itself as through mediating professionals and institutions. In the civilization theory this control is chiefly considered to be a consequence of the civilization pressure citizens increasingly exert on one another, whereby professional regimes play a mainly intermediary part. Theoreticians such as Foucault and Donzelot stress the position of power these regimes have obtained by creating new, ostensibly neutral containment techniques. In their opinion, new forms of population control have come into being in this process of modernization. In contrast to the past, these are not immediately punitive and oppressive, but aim rather at subtle adaptation and treatment. According to Van Lieshout (1993) this picture should at least be filled out; both experts and lay people have become increasingly focused on problems and potential problems. In the presentation of problems the ideas of the two groups have become interwoven. The specific mechanisms of generalization, individualization and assigning effects are entirely in line with this problem culture. They not only presuppose professionals and institutions that are actively problematizing, but also a public that endorse their definitions of problems.

The net effect of the processes described here is that in our society children and young people are looked upon more and more as constituting a (potential) problem. As we have already seen, the phenomenon manifests itself all the more forcefully in regard to disadvantaged or minority groups. This problematization is harmful, both for the self-image and identity formation of young people and for society as a whole. The perception of young people as a problem as well as the actual policy measures based on this have gradually become so dominant that we are hard put to face up to their positive potential. On the one hand there is a danger that a negative educational climate is created, in which young people do not sufficiently get the feeling that they are appreciated as present and future members of society. On the other hand the tangible contributions young people are able to make to society are insufficiently used and respected. These are the reasons for our endeavour, in the next chapter, to develop an alternative to this perspective. From 'youth as a problem' to 'youth as potential'.

References

Abma R (1986) Cultuur en tegencultuur in het Nederlands jeugdonderzoek. In: M Matthijssen e.a. (red) *Beelden van jeugd*. Groningen: Wolters Noordhof. pp. 209–29.

Ariès Ph (1987) *De ontdekking van het kind. Sociale geschiedenis van school en gezin*. Amsterdam: Bert Bakker. (Oorspronkelijke uitgave 1960.)

Bogt T ter & C van Praag (1992) *Jongeren op de drempel van de jaren negentig*. 's-Gravenhage/Rijswijk, VUGA/SCP.

Bosga M (1993) *Samenwerking in ontwikkeling (2). Achtergrondstudie over de VTO-ondersteuningsfuncties*. Zoetermeer: Nationale Raad voor de Volksgezondheid/Universiteit Utrecht.

Bronfenbrenner U (1979) *The ecology of human development*. Cambridge, Mass: Harvard University Press.

DeMause L (1974) *The history of childhood*. New York: Psychohistory Press.

Diekstra RFW (1992) De adolescentie: biologische, psychologische en sociale aspecten. In: RFW Diekstra (ed) *Jeugd in ontwikkeling*. 's-Gravenhage: SDU. pp. 111–57.

Diekstra RFW (1993) Opvoeding tot opvoeden: ontwikkeling en overheidsbeleid. *Jeugd en Samenleving* 6/7. pp. 309–29.

Dieleman AJ & AC Perreijn (1993) Inleiding. In: AJ Dieleman, FJ van der Linden & AC Perreijn (red) *Jeugd in Meervoud*. Utrecht/Heerlen: Tijdstroom & Open Universiteit. pp. 15–34.

Donzelot J (1979) *The policing of families*. New York: Pantheon.

Elias N (1982) *Het civilisatieproces. Sociogenetische en psychogenetische onderzoekingen*, deel 1 en 2. Utrecht: Spectrum.

Foucault M (1975) *Surveillir et punir: la naissance de la prison*. Parijs: Gallimard.

Halsema F & R Coppes (1993) Politici roepen maar wat over criminele jeugd. *Volkskrant*, 25-3-1993. p. 11.

Heemskerk J (1993) Negatief beeld van jeugdigen berust op vooroordelen. *Volkskrant*, 5-5-1993.

Helder M (1993) Column. *Volkskrant*, 19-3-1993.

Junger-Tas J (1993) Normen, waarden en jeugdcriminaliteit. *CDA-Actueel* 24-6-1993.

Laan PH van der (1993) Is het waar? Over jeugddelinquentie en strafrechtelijke reacties. *FJR*, nr. 10. pp. 223–9.

Lalonde M (1974) *A new perspective on the health of the Canadians*. Ottawa: Ministry of National Health and Welfare.

Lieshout I van (1993) *Deskundigen en ouders van nu. Bindingen in een probleemcultuur*. Dissertatie Universiteit Utrecht. Utrecht: De Tijdstroom.

Meeus W (1993) Jeugd en jeugdonderzoek in Nederland. De betekenis van 'Jongeren op de drempel van de jaren negentig' en 'Jeugd in Ontwikkeling' voor de kennis over de jeugd. *Jeugd en Samenleving*, 6/7. pp. 330–41.

Ministerie van Justitie (1992) *Verslag expert-meeting sociaal-normatieve opvoeding*, 7-4-1992.

Ministerie van Welzijn, Volksgezondheid en Cultuur (1992) *Rapportage meisjesbeleid, Op weg naar integratie*. 's-Gravenhage: WVC.

Ministerie van Welzijn, Volksgezondheid en Cultuur (1993) *Jeugd verdient de toekomst. Nota intersectoraal jeugdbeleid.* 's-Gravenhage: WVC.

Noordman J & H van Setten (1989) De ontwikkeling van de ouder/kind-verhouding in het gezin. In: HFM Peeters, L Dresen-Coenders & T Brandenburg (red) *Vijf eeuwen gezinsleven. Liefde, huwelijk en opvoeding in Nederland.* Nijmegen: SUN. pp. 140–62.

Peeters HFM (1975) *Kind en jeugdige in het begin van de moderne tijd.* Meppel: Boom. (oorspr. uitg. 1966.)

Pollock LA (1983) *Forgotten children. Parent–child relations from 1500 to 1900.* Cambridge: Cambridge University Press.

Praag C van (1993) Hoe gaat het met de jeugd? Een kleine speurtocht naar ongerief. *Jeugd en Samenleving,* 6/7. pp. 292–308.

Raad voor het Jeugdbeleid (1994) *Aanval op uitval.* Bestrijding van uitval van jeugdigen. Utrecht: SWP.

Röling HQ (1982) Gezinsgeschiedenis en gezinsideologie. In: B Kruithof, J Noordman & P de Rooy (red) *Geschiedenis van opvoeding en onderwijs.* Inleiding bronnenonderzoek. pp. 37–66. Nijmegen: SUN.

Roos JPH & REX Boswinkel (1981) Het geminachte kind. Een historisch perspectief. *Intermediair,* jrg. 17, 20 mrt. pp. 21–7.

Sameroff AJ (1975) Early influences on development: Fact or fancy. *Merill Palmer Quarterly,* Vol. 21, nr. 4. pp. 267–94.

Schnabel P (1992) Het kostbare kind. Reflecties bij de eeuw van het kind. *Tijdschrift voor Kindergeneeskunde,* jrg. 60, nr.4. pp. 91–7.

Spiecker B & F Groenendijk (1980) Wat is er met het kind gebeurd? Het effect-ontwikkelingsmodel en de geschiedenis van het kind. *Pedagogische Studiën,* 57. pp. 1–10.

Swaan A de (1989) *Zorg en de Staat. Welzijn, onderwijs en gezondheidszorg in Europa en de Verenigde Staten in de nieuwe tijd.* Amsterdam: Bert Bakker.

Winter M de (1986) *Het voorspelbare kind.* VTO *(vroegtijdige onderkenning van ontwikkelingsstoornissen) in wetenschappelijk en sociaal-historisch perspectief.* Lisse: Swets & Zeitlinger. Dissertatie Katholieke Universiteit Brabant.

Winter M de (1992) Preventiekinderen. In: A. Hol (red) *Opvoedingson-dersteuning.* Utrecht: SWP. pp. 56–63.

Witte R & Y Yesilgöz (1992) Ethnische minderheden: "misdadige crimina-lisering". *LBR Bulletin,* nr. 4. pp. 21–3.

Zijderveld AC (1992) *Normvervaging, een cultuursociologische notitie.* zie: Ministerie van justitie 1992: expert-meeting sociaal-normatieve opvoeding.

Participating fellow citizens

Introduction

As brought forward in the previous chapter, the creation in and by society of images of children and young people is dominated by problems. Both youth policy and research in this field are in the same spirit. Yet there are interesting hiatuses in this problem argument. In the first place the inclination to see problems is not equally strong in all sections of society. For instance in the school system, the stimulation of development and social opportunities is a far more important aim than the recognition and prevention of problems, though even in this field the culture of problems seems to be gaining ground with the extension of care and the stronger educational assignment (cf. Chapter 5). In local youth policy moreover, we discern a cautious, but successful tendency to address the qualities and potential of young people rather than their difficulties. In the second place it remains to be seen in how far children and youngsters will let themselves be problematized. In general this is hard to forecast but looking, for instance, at the results of the study 'Social environments of children up to the age of 12 in the Netherlands', we do not get the impression that we are faced with a dejected generation[1] (Peeters & Woldringh, 1993). This picture is confirmed in a comparable study into the social environments of young people between 12 and 21 years old, which shows that the great majority (the by now familiar 80%) is happy with the situation at home, with the group of friends, and at school (van der Linden, 1990). Without wanting to play down real problems, the mirror held up to us by young people in such research may well constitute a major stimulus to move with the times in this regard. In the third place a growing number of researchers and policy makers are coming to the conclusion that problematization has run its course. In the previous chapter youth researcher Meeus was quoted as concluding that scientific research itself made a considerable contribution to the creation of the legend of youth as a problem (Meeus, 1993). The government memorandum 'Youth deserves the future' warns against potentially stigmatizing effects that may result from a youth policy with a

---

[1] It should be noted that those questioned were mainly educators. Out of the target group of this study, only the oldest children were asked to answer a questionnaire themselves. Overall the study presents a rather optimistic view of the way education is experienced, at least by parents: 44% think their children are (very) easy; 49% judge them to be 'ordinary', that is to say with 'normal little problems'; and 7% say that they generally find it 'hard' to 'very hard' to cope with their children.

bias towards problems (Ministry of Welfare, Public Health and Cultural Affairs WVC, 1993).

The image of 'youth as a problem' obviously displays notable weak spots: it is only very partially based on factual data, it shows a self-fulfilling tendency, it disregards the advantages a non-problematizing approach may have both for young people themselves and for society. But the major disadvantage is certainly the negation of the capabilities young people have and their need to exercise these. At the same time the outlines of a competing approach are appearing; by this we mean social attitudes and practice in which children and youngsters are primarily addressed on the basis of their present and potential capabilities and their need for these to be recognized and developed, rather than on the basis of their problems and shortcomings. Naturally such a reversal in thought and action regarding young people does not come about at the drop of a hat. After all, such replacement of a paradigm severely affects the functioning of various social sectors, institutions and persons dealing with children and youngsters. The core concepts connected with this metamorphosis are citizenship and participation. In practice this comes down to regarding children and youngsters as fellow citizens, people whose share in society is appreciated and stimulated because of the constructive contribution they are able to make. Participation, which we may provisionally define as *opportunities for children and young people to be actively involved in (the decision making on) their own living environment* is a major condition.

In this chapter we first elaborate the theory of these two concepts. We consider the relationship between the participation and citizenship of adults and the young, and on what conditions the two concepts can be tailored to fit young people. Subsequently we examine the role of participating citizenship in social policy regarding the young, at a national as well as an international level.

What is participation?

The word participation may be used in both passive and active senses. Here we use the word in the active sense. As far as young people are concerned we are emphatically not discussing participation in family activities, sports clubs and youth organizations, in training or work, in other words, in activities organized for the benefit of young people. What it is all about is shared responsibility and active engagement, the core elements of an approach in which the competence of the individual is addressed. Usually a distinction is made between participation in a political sense and in a social form. Castenmiller (1989, page 62) defines political participation as 'the behaviour of citizens aimed at influencing the political decision-making process directly or indirectly'. Social participation is not much concerned with formal political processes, but with influencing policy that affects daily life in a direct way, for instance at neighbourhood level or involving educational institutions or work situations (cf. van der Kooy, 1989).

Since the 1960s active social participation by *adults* has become a major social and political theme in many western countries. This was connected with the democratization process, in which diverse groups claimed a greater voice in the decision-making that affected their own interests. Well-known examples of this are the groups of inhabitants in inner city areas who insisted on public consultation in cases of renovation, and the patients' associations which from the 1970s have demanded influence to counteract abuses in psychiatric practice. During this period Bills were introduced in the Netherlands establishing the democratization of welfare organizations and of the universities, and mandatory works councils. At provincial and local levels procedures were developed for public consultation in regional planning, key decisions in urban and rural planning, town rehabilitation and traffic. Developments are taking place in health care and education which indicate a growing (albeit sometimes very gradual) influence of patients, and of parents and pupils. In institutional health care especially there are often councils of inmates or patients, while general and specific organizations of patients are becoming an ever more powerful factor in the national health policy. For schools there are statutory regulations for the consultation of parents, pupils and staff, even if their influence – particularly of the pupils – on school policy is still very marginal. By the end of the 1980s we see a renewed interest in public participation in many countries. The authorities wanted to reduce the gap between institutions and the public by decentralizing authority and funding, so that the population could be more closely involved in caring for the liveability of their own environment. Besides that, extra attention was paid to the education of disadvantaged groups in order to enhance their chances of employment and to counteract marginalization. Social participation by children and young people contrasts sharply with these developments concerning participation by adults – even though many are, rightly, far from content with the extent to which this takes place.

Children's participation: a first investigation

The American psychologist Roger Hart carried out an international study for UNICEF on children's participation. He defines participation as the 'fundamental right of citizenship ... referring generally to the process of sharing decisions which affect one's life and the life of the community in which one lives. It is the means by which a democracy is built and it is a standard against which democracies should be measured' (Hart, 1992, page 5). He finds that the importance of participation of children and young people 'is a subject of strongly divergent opinion'. Opinions vary from 'children should be protected from such adult responsibilities' to 'children's participation is the very source of social change'. He mentions two main arguments for children's participation. Firstly he considers it necessary from the perspective of developmental psychology: 'It is unrealistic to expect them suddenly to become responsible, participating adults at the age of 16, 18 or 21 without prior exposure to the skills and responsibilities involved'. Secondly children's participation, as indicated by his extensive international documentation, appears to be able to play a significant part in community development. Actively involving children in the improvement of their own living environment may be a catalyst that activates a local community as a whole.

In a Council of Europe report on local youth policy, youth participation is defined as 'young people's right to be included, to be allowed and encouraged to assume duties and responsibilities and to make one's own decisions' (Council of Europe, 1993). The Council elaborates on this right to take part in society and the responsibilities towards it in two specific ways: participation means the right to influence in a democratic manner processes bearing upon one's own life, and to be involved in the development of local youth policy. Although this definition does not in fact deviate very much from Hart's, the emphasis in the two reports is clearly different. Whereas Hart notably stresses the aspects of democratic education, in the European report strengthening the power of young people plays a crucial part. The report even rejects as dangerous an educational youth policy that does not immediately result in the enlargement of the material social influence of young people. It emphatically points out the risk that youth participation is made use of to integrate young people into existing social structures on which they are then unable to exert any influence at all. One example was in the former Soviet Union, where participation in the only youth organization allowed (Komsomol) was a means to socialize youth according to the principles of the communist system. In Nazi Germany the Hitler-Jugend worked on the same principle. But participation may also be used in far less extreme and direct ways to make young people toe the line; in other words, to neutralize their power. Referring to Foucault, the report alleges that 'hidden curricula' with disciplinary and normalizing effects often play a part in youth policy. It is not uncommon that organized leisure activities for young people have an implicit aim to foster morality and good behaviour. This is the very process the writers of the European report want to abandon, because in the first place it appeals especially to the moral panic and society's fears about young people (cf. Cohen, 1972), and in the second place because it produces a type of young people that is robbed of its social and cultural creativity (cf.

Willis, 1990). The consequences of this approach can be seen among the East-European young who grew up under a regime of disciplinary participation. To them, every form of youth policy is suspect and reprehensible (Council of Europe, 1993, page 8). Genuine participation therefore, according to the writers of the European report, implies the granting of material influence to young people: influence on the way in which they organize their own lives, on the conditions of their lives and on the policy that is pursued towards them. The pedagogic perspective at the basis of this power approach has been notably inspired by the work of Paulo Freire. Youth is one of the oppressed groups in capitalist society that is to be liberated by way of participation. Obtaining insight into and power over one's own reality is the starting point (cf. Freire, 1972).

There are two reasons for these aims of participation: education in democracy and strengthening of young people's position of power, appearing here as opposites. In the first place the UNICEF report relates to the age group up to the age of 18, therefore including young children. Conversely the Council of Europe report is mainly about the position of older youth, which is usually taken to refer to the age group between 12 and 25 years of age. It will be clear that social influence becomes a more important factor as the age of those involved rises. In the second place there is the problem that the two reports proclaim their visions on the participation of the young without clearly relating these to young people's position in society, their rights and needs. In this way the discussion on participation quickly takes on a moralistic and ideological character: education versus power, emancipation versus discipline. To prevent this the notion should be linked to the actual social context in which young people live, and which, as we know, may vary greatly in different parts of the world. In the following sections we first consider the changing practice of citizenship as a context for children's participation in society.

Citizenship

In the last few years the relation between the state and its citizens has become a major discussion theme in western welfare states. Authorities and politicians complain about calculating citizens who think of the state as a lucky dip, about a dwindling sense of values and about a declining sense of collective responsibility. Citizens on the other hand feel inadequately protected by the state (from crime for instance), plagued by bureaucracy and regulations, and they become frustrated by the inaccessibility of public authorities. Usually the cause of this growing gap is sought in processes such as individualization and the breaking down of old barriers, basically religious and social ones, with, in consequence, the disappearance of the old socially prescriptive framework. Sometimes the citizen is blamed because of his calculating attitude, sometimes the state because of its bureaucratic disposition.

The notion of citizenship plays a prominent part in discussions on these matters. Although this notion daunts many people because of its former connotation of conservatism, it is nowadays used in various versions to describe and construe (desirable) relations between individual and society. Dahrendorf describes citizenship as 'a collection of entitlements common to all members of society' (Dahrendorf, 1988). Entitlements are 'rights meant to be protected from the vagaries of day to day politics', and may be broken down into political and social civil rights. Suffrage and eligibility, freedom of speech and the right of assembly are examples of the former; access to social services, health services and to education of the latter. In Dahrendorf's scenario, young children and those people who have had to be temporarily deprived of their citizenship because of mental illness or criminal behaviour are excluded from political rights. Their civil rights mainly consist of the right to be protected from exploitation and abuse. Against these entitlements there are duties, such as paying taxes and staying within the law. These apply in general to all citizens, yet 'apprentice citizens' pose a problem in this respect: they are minors but nevertheless responsible for a number of serious crimes (Dahrendorf, ibid., page 7). In a study by the Dutch Scientific Advisory Board on Government Policy (WRR) the contemporary citizen is typified as 'someone who plays the twin roles of governing and being governed in an autonomous, judicious and loyal way' (van Gunsteren, 1992). It is in these very twin roles that the essence of the civil society[2] is to be found: the citizens' state. Ultimately, such a society can exist only if on the one hand people are loyal to the rules jointly established (the consensus for instance on the government monopoly of violence, and on the right to diversity), and on the other hand if they are actively, critically and autonomously involved in the functioning of the community. The latter ideal makes a strong demand on the competence of the modern citizen. His or her repertoire includes 'debate, reasonableness, democracy', as well as 'sensible, competent and responsible handling of authority, situations and positions of power' (van Gunsteren, ibid., page 18). The picture of the citizen as a key figure of modern society is completed by tolerance and respect for diversity of identities, opinions and behaviour (plurality); the readiness to bear responsibility in one's own environment, in groups, organizations and political structures; and finally the willingness to take a stand when principles of the civil society are at stake (citizenship as a reserve circuit).

These opinions however, are often subject to criticism. If citizenship and

---

[2]The WRR report here uses the term 'republic'.

public spirit were rather obvious and commonly held political ideals up to the mid-1960s, in the 1970s and 1980s the 'standard citizen' is unmasked step by step (Hartman, 1989). First as a capitalist (citizenship conceals class differences), then as a man (citizenship conceals the inequality of power between the sexes), subsequently as white (citizenship discriminates on the basis of ethnic origins) and finally as a provider (marginalization of economically inactive persons impedes access to active citizenship). In short, citizenship has been fragmented into a great diversity of interests of differing groups and categories, which have come to be in a competitive situation with one another[3]. Consequently, in the modern social arena, groups of citizens, usually aided and abetted by professionals with a vested interest, are more often to be seen in combat with one another for the favour of authorities and politicians. The competition between different patients' associations in health care is a good example (cf. de Winter, 1986). The culture of problems plays a major part in this competition: the articulation of suffering proves to be a good tool for the promotion of interests. A weak spot in the exposition of the neo-republican citizen (as van Gunsteren refers to his ideal) is the situation of people who for some reason find themselves in a position of dependence. This applies for instance to women without an independent income, to those incapacitated for work, to the chronically ill and the handicapped, and naturally to children and young people. The very standard of independence inherent in modern citizenship contributes to social marginalization of these groups. In modern society independence has increasingly come to mean economic independence; earning one's own salary. Anyone who does not meet this standard, for instance because he or she is a carer, is in care or is growing up, loses social status and influence; in other words is a second-class citizen (cf. Parlevliet & Sevenhuijsen, 1992). Feminist critics of the liberal-individualist civic ideal assert that citizenship and its associated rights derive from an atomistic portrayal of humankind. The citizen is a separate individual who is primarily pursuing his personal interests, in competition with others, and is continuously claiming personal rights. An ideology of this type has no room for values and considerations such as solidarity, care, compassion and affection (Held, in Sevenhuijsen, 1993). Yet we are gradually seeing some recognition of the importance of such a care ethic as an element of citizenship. In the Netherlands nowadays people speak of a threefold perspective for the future: boys and girls must be prepared for economic independence (i.e. paid work), for tasks of caring (i.e. unpaid

---

[3]As a counterweight to the continuing fragmentation, Hartman advocates a reconsideration of the old civic ideal along four lines: (1) next to the emphasis on specific interests the common (i.e. shared) values and the collective adherence to the democratic system should receive more attention; (2) the citizen should more often be addressed as an individual, his independent judgement should be fostered; (3) duties as well as rights should be stressed; (4) social organizations which give citizens a certain independence from the state should be strengthened (Hartman, ibid., pages 30–31).

work) and for social participation in other sectors (Raad voor het jeugdbeleid, 1991, 1992). The introduction of care as a school subject in the lower forms of secondary education is a first, albeit cautious step.

The plea for active citizenship is the socio-political context guiding social commitment and participation. The various points of view in this debate demonstrate a number of shared ideals such as a democratic outlook, responsibility, autonomy, plurality and respect for the integrity of others. On the other hand citizenship proves to work as a social dividing line; between active and inactive people, between the powerful and the powerless and, significant in this context, between adults and the young. To avert the danger of stigmatization and exclusion, the American political scientist, I.M. Young, deems empowerment necessary: a process in which 'individual, relatively powerless persons dialogue with each other and thereby come to understand the social sources of their powerlessness, and see the possibility of acting collectively to change their social environment' (Young, 1992)[4].

Children and citizenship

When we try to apply the concept of citizenship to children, we are faced with a number of problems. The most fundamental question is whether or not children are citizens anyway. There seems to be fairly general consensus in the political sense of the word. In Dahrendorf's words: children are in the company of lunatics and criminals in being excluded from active political civil rights, but have all the more right to basic provisions and protection. Even in Hartman's exposure of the myth of citizenship the negation of the citizen solely as an adult is conspicuously absent. Young people then are not citizens in the formal political sense of the word. Only at the age of 18 do they have the right to vote, only then can they formally take part in government. Now and then dissenting opinions are heard from some representatives of the movement for children's rights. Recently, for instance, there was a plea to give minors the right to vote (Franklin, cited by van Nijnatten, 1993).

The citizenship of children and young people in the social and legal sense is the subject of much more discussion. On the basis of an extensive international comparative study into the rights and position of children, Veerman (1992) concludes that since the beginning of this century major

---

[4]An identical opinion to that met in the definition of youth participation by the Council of Europe.

changes have occurred in the way in which they are approached socially. From being deserving cases and objects of protection (objects of rights), children have become persons vested with rights (subjects of rights): their opinions are more often expressed, asked for and respected. In this period young people's interests have been socialized: whereas for a long time their defence was the business of benevolent, charitably inclined individuals, nowadays in many countries this is the responsibility of political and social institutions. This is by no means to say that children's rights are unvaryingly ensured everywhere, or even in the Netherlands. For instance, in the Netherlands, legal access specifically for children as well as ombudsmen for children by which 'conditions are created for children to stand up for themselves and realize their rights' (de Langen, 1991 a,b) have been advocated for a considerable time. However, there are also those who warn against the negative effects of bringing children's lives even further into the legal sphere. van Nijnatten (1993) points out the danger that too much emphasis on the legal position of youngsters could cause other factors influencing their life–world to be neglected. More rights may after all lead to partial loss of protection, since young people are then deemed to be capable of pursuing these rights (ibid., page 12). Veerman criticizes the 'Kiddy Libbers' (the American nickname for the children's rights movement), because just wanting to grant children equal power and rights ignores their as yet restricted possibilities. 'It is our opinion that the unlimited rights the Kiddy Libbers want to give to children withhold from them the most essential right: to be a child' says Veerman (ibid., page 937). So it appears that what is in children's interest, is far from being an objective quantity which adults can establish universally for all children. Sevenhuijsen for this reason argues for restraint as far as the translation of children's interests into rights are concerned. She deems it important to 'create social and political space in which children can speak for themselves, not in the name of a common children's interest, but rather as an opportunity to bring their specific needs and problems to the fore' (Sevenhuijsen, 1993, page 56). Such comments uncover another dilemma in the theories on children and citizenship. To what extent can we expect autonomy, independence and responsibility of young people, whereas their age, their development and their world, on the contrary, presuppose dependence, inequality, trust in adults and intimacy? Present and future citizens are increasingly expected to be committed to, and to participate in, society, but at the same time there seem to be hardly any possibilities for children and young people to familiarize themselves with these tasks. 'Practising democratic decision-making' for instance, can be found in hardly any educational curriculum. This makes it clear that there is a need to develop an *intermediate area for the development of citizenship*. The German pedagogue Klaus Mollenhauer (1986) draws attention to the high-tension area in which the development to adult citizenship takes place: 'as the social world becomes more complex, so do the relationships within that world become less accessible for the child, who nevertheless will have to live with these relationships in the future. And the more complex the social world becomes, the less he will be able to find whatever he needs for his future in his primary life–world' (ibid., page 20).

In short, young people have a great deal to learn about citizenship, so that an educational approach is at least as important as a strictly political and legal one. The question of whether they are citizens can really be compared to the question of whether they are adults. If citizenship is a social ideal, young people are citizens in the making, and they should be treated as such. That is to say they should be given the opportunity to develop gradually into committed, autonomous, discerning and responsible members of the community. For that very reason they need the social space to learn to formulate their specific needs, ideas and problems themselves, which means that they need an environment that provides the support as well as the conditions. Then another question presents itself, namely whether young people actually want to be or become citizens? What if, for instance, they are absolutely disinclined to be loyal to the community? Many of their parents are equally disinclined and will undoubtedly pass on this attitude; others to the contrary may have very 'bourgeois' parents against whom they are just going into opposition. Naturally the material conditions people live in and their expectations about the future play an important part in an attitude towards citizenship, of parents and children alike. If parents are in a dead-end situation, perhaps because of long-time unemployment and poverty, or if young people lack the perspective of good further education or satisfying paid work, modern ideals about citizenship will certainly not fall on fertile ground. In such situations after all, people rightly feel that fundamental rights of citizenship are not being afforded (cf. Dahrendorf, page 30). So it is very likely that the associated duties will not be experienced as such either. Citizenship therefore remains a vague illusion if conditions are not created for an acceptable perspective. Notwithstanding this essential observation an educational stance remains crucial; young persons have the right to determine their own future. However, as Mollenhauer puts it: 'they can only conceive this within the context of the pattern of life adults present them with' (Mollenhauer, 1986, page 18). In other words, society has an obligation towards young people to formulate its own cultural content and its values for the future, however diverse these may be, and to propagate these in education. Even if this should do no more than provide young people with an opportunity to acquire an autonomous position towards such content and values.

In conclusion: a society wishing to pursue an active citizenship ideal is faced with a social and educational challenge. Children and young people are citizens in the making, and should therefore be given the opportunity to develop that citizenship. In this respect it is important in the first place that some fundamental material conditions are met: the citizenship entitlements should have some reality, also for children and young people. Without the perspective of sufficient opportunities for development, for instance in the shape of a good education and chances of paid employment, and without experiencing that their rights are respected, few young people will be inclined to bother about the duties involved in citizenship. In the second place social space is necessary for the development of citizenship, space in which the required competence and attitudes can be learned and practised by trial and error. Participation is an essential means to this: on the one hand it contributes to the empowerment of young people, by which they themselves learn to articulate their social needs; on the other hand it is a major instrument in training values and capacities required in the framework of modern citizenship. In this respect it is not only criteria such as independent judgement, responsibility and loyalty that are at stake, but also values which can be classified as care-ethics: solidarity, care and affection. This citizenship concept of course implies the competence and freedom to take up an independent position oneself, even regarding the ideal of citizenship itself. A condition however is that this ideal is presented live to young people. Gradually such a perspective is receiving some international recognition. In the UN Convention on the Rights of the Child participation has even been established as a civil right, albeit with certain restrictions.

The UN Convention on the Rights of the Child

In 1990, after ten years of laborious negotiations, the UN Convention on the Rights of the Child came into effect. Besides articles on provisions and protection for children (defined as every human being below the age of 18 years), this Convention, for the first time in the history of international human rights conventions, comprises a number of obligations on the right of participation by young people. The Articles concerned are[5]:

- *Article 12*: Right to express views in matters affecting the child

- *Article 13*: Right to freedom of expression (general)

- *Article 14*: Right to freedom of thought, conscience and religion

- *Article 15*: Right to freedom of association and assembly

- *Article 30*: Right of children of minority communities and indigenous populations to enjoy their own culture and to practice their own religion.

---

[5]For a full overview of the Convention Articles see: Ling (1993).

Although these rights to freedoms are very basic in our eyes, so that for the situation in many western countries they seem to have little added value, they are of great importance internationally. They define children as independent persons vested with rights, to whom active participation in society is as important as care and protection. This means that children may invoke it, but also that adults, and especially authorities, have a duty to create the conditions. Article 12 reads:

> *States' parties shall assure to the child who is capable of forming his or her own views the right to express those views freely in all matters affecting the child, the views of the child being given due weight in accordance with the age and maturity of the child.*

> *For this purpose, the child shall in particular be provided the opportunity to be heard in any judicial and administrative proceedings affecting the child, either directly, or through a representative or an appropriate body, in a manner consistent with the procedural rules of national law.*

Article 13 goes a step further, but at the same time includes a number of restrictions and escape clauses:

> *The child shall have the right to freedom of expression; this right shall include freedom to seek, receive and impart information and ideas of all kinds, regardless of frontiers, either orally, in writing or in print, in the form of art, or through any other media of the child's choice.*

> *The exercise of this right may be subject to certain restrictions, but these shall only be such as are provided by law and are necessary:*

> *(a) for respect of the rights or reputations of others; or*

> *(b) for the protection of national security or of public order, or of public health and morals.*

Such phrasing forms the impression of it resulting from laboriously reached compromises. Indeed, the rights to freedom of thought, conscience and religion (Article 14) and the right to freedom of association and assembly (Article 15) are similarly restricted. Notably Article 14 has given rise to great resistance, Veerman even qualifying it as one of the most controversial of the whole Convention (Veerman, 1992, page 194). A number of Islamic countries contested the freedom of religion, because it is at odds with the tradition that children adopt the religion of their parents. During the discussions delegates from the Soviet Union, Algeria, China, Iraq and Poland rejected the freedom of association and assembly for reasons that can easily be surmised. Nevertheless the Convention has now been ratified by over 150 countries. In how far the situation of children whose civil rights are grossly violated will be affected by this ratification is, of course, still far from clear[6]. However, the text of the Convention establishes some clear boundaries, rights and duties. With it the active involvement of children in international society has become one of the fundamental human rights. This is not to say that numerous countries have developed an active policy on children's participation; hardly any are mentioned in UNICEF or Council of Europe reports.

Participation in Dutch youth policy

Young people's participation is a concept that has been used to an extremely varying extent, but also in extremely fluctuating senses in Dutch youth policy since the Second World War. From an analysis of the contents of policy documents about young people[7] published between 1945 and 1990 Voortman (1991) concludes that 'participation' is in fact used in three different ways. Between 1945 and 1960, a period in which the responsibility for youth policy mainly lay with private initiatives and the government's role was restricted to providing subsidies, *fitting young people into society* was the central theme. This was the period when the 'unruliness of the mass of youth' was a cause for concern to many people, and when participation, if the term was used at all, aimed to turn these young people into 'community members'. Attention was paid notably to the provision of sufficient kinds of proper leisure activities through independent youth work. In the second half of the 1960s the interest in participation, notably in the sense of *consultation and participation in decision-making,* increased greatly. Youth policy was no longer dominated by unruliness, but far more by youth discontent about, and resistance to, the established order of the grown-ups. On the one hand more notice had be taken of the desires and needs of young people themselves, on the other their influence on society had to be strengthened. In this context the Dutch Ministry of Social Work in 1969 advocated the promotion of participation in decision-making through the establishment of local youth policy boards. In the course of the seventies the accent shifts more and more towards *formative education.* Participation becomes a means to personal development and self-expression: 'young people should have the opportunity to develop their own ideas, to bear responsibility themselves and learn to make their own choices with regard to their future society' as a policy memorandum from

---

[6]Serious doubts on this subject have been expressed in two reports on the human rights situation of children in Guatemala. These rights appear still to be violated in a gross and extremely violent manner, notwithstanding the fact that the country was one of the first to ratify the UN Convention (see Onvlee, 1992).

[7]Defined in the study as 'young people between 12 and 25 years old'.

1975 states. In fact this trend towards formative education continues into the middle of the 1980s, but at an earlier date attention already shifts from youth policy to specific problem groups: young people in multiple disadvantaged situations. Gradually participation as a theme of policy fades, since people clearly prefer other 'measures to keep these youngsters in check' (Voortman, ibid., page 56).

From 1990 the participation of young people makes a strong comeback in government policy. In her policy letter, 'Cooperating in new ways', the Minister of Welfare, Public Health and Cultural Affairs (WVC) outlines her intentions for welfare policy in the 1990s (Ministry of WVC, 1991). In line with social renewal, then reigning supreme, the crux is 'to strengthen and maintain independence'. 'People should be protected', the Minister writes, 'from finding themselves in a downward spiral of marginalization and minority formation, and from ending up in a hopeless situation, characterized by social isolation and substantial dependence on all kinds of provisions. Such processes can be interrupted by activating people's vital potential and promoting integration'. This intention was then elaborated in regard to young people, namely in the policy document 'Youth deserves the future' (Ministry of WVC, 1993a). In it the main aims for integrated youth policy are named as 'promoting opportunities' and 'preventing and tackling dropping out among young people'. Although the appeal to young people's own competence is presented as a general policy vision (and therefore applicable to all young people), in the elaboration the accent is strongly on young people with problems. In this way participation acquires a mainly *preventive function*. Commitment to, and taking an active part in society and its structures stimulates problem resolving competence, and prevents young people from being marginalized. The document also calls for special attention to be paid to young people in high-risk situations: children from isolated families, some young people from ethnic minorities and girls who have had little education (Ministry of WVC, 1993b).

In this policy the attentive reader will recognize each of the three meanings of participation mentioned before: fitting in, consultation and formative education. What is new is that these elements have been linked in a modern prevention strategy. Strengthening citizenship, in this case the right of young people to be consulted, to be well provided with information, to a good education, to care and support, and to respect from adults, is considered an important means to halt the 'problems young people have and cause', as well as to cut back on public spending. The document states: 'young people are precious in more than one respect, figuratively because they are becoming scarce (due to double degreeing and the growing number of the elderly); literally because society invests heavily in schooling and further education, and sees day-by-day how expensive it is to re-introduce into society young people who drop out or are threatening to drop out' (Ministry of WVC, 1993a, page 34). This is a legitimate point of view as such, but it conceals a patent risk. Participation of young people is not in this case defined as an absolute, but as an instrumental (and therefore relative) requirement. Active commitment is advocated because of its preventive potential, whereas in principle a basic need as well as a basic right are at stake. In this way youth as well as society remain captive in the culture of problems mentioned before. Thus citizenship in the making runs the risk of becoming or remaining a cyclically sensitive quantity. The history of children, but also their present position in many parts of the world, prove how dangerous such dependence is. Participation by children and young people may well have preventive and socio-economic effects – so much the better – but it should be pursued independently of these as an absolute principle of a democratic society.

Levels of participation

The UNICEF report quoted earlier gives numerous examples of children's participation projects, underway all over the world (Hart, 1992). The overview demonstrates an enormous variety as to character, content and organization of such projects. They vary from local 'trade unions' of Philippine street children and a national organization of Brazilian street children, to American children who have themselves designed and introduced an observation of behaviour system for their class. This variety also demonstrates the degree to which the significance of children's participation depends on the social context in which it takes place. Whereas projects that NGOs (non-governmental organizations) set up for street children and vagrant children in Third World countries are in the first place aimed at the fundamental conditions for existence, namely strengthening their socio-economic situation and their social safety (empowerment), children's participation in western countries envisages education for citizenship through consultation and democratic education. It is therefore not a good idea to compare such projects without taking into account the social function each has. It also becomes clear that the concept of children's participation, and the right to it, remains fairly gratuitous if its aims are not clearly defined. However strange it may sound, in some cases assigning the label of 'children's participation' appears to serve well to restrict children's involvement. In other words, the concept needs to be further differentiated. For this purpose, Hart, analogous to a classification by Arnstein (1969), devised his ladder of participation. The first three steps embrace forms of apparent participation, that is activities in which children do indeed figure, but on which they cannot exert substantial influence. These are, however, worth mentioning, because they are frequently found practices in which the involvement of children, for whatever reason, is simulated. They are:

1 *Manipulation*: children are engaged or used for the benefit of their own
   interests, formulated by adults, while the children themselves do not
   understand the implications. For example: toddlers carrying banners in
   a demonstration for family allowances, or making drawings of a
   playground of which no practical use is made in its design.

2 *Decoration*: children are called in to embellish adult actions, for
   instance by song, dance and other affecting activities. Adults do not,
   however, pretend that all this is in the interests of the children
   themselves.

3 *Tokenism*: Children are apparently given a voice, but this is to serve the
   child-friendly image adults want to create rather than the interest of the
   children themselves. According to Hart (1992) this is common practice,
   notably in the western world, for instance on conference panels, where
   the radiating charm of children often makes a great impression.

Real participation by children begins on rung four of the ladder, wherever
they are given sufficient insight into the intentions of a certain project or
activity. The greater the extent of own initiative and freedom of choice, the
higher the classification on the ladder of participation (rungs four to eight).

4 *Assigned but informed*: adults take the initiative to call in children, but
   inform them on how and why. Only after the children have come to
   understand the intentions of the project and the point of their
   involvement (see Hart, page 12) do the children decide whether or
   not to take part. Hart gives the example of bringing in children as
   'pages' of 71 government leaders during the World Summit for
   Children, a meeting dealing with the rights of the child. One of the
   aims of the permanent presence of children during the conference was
   to compel the leaders to take substantial steps.

5 *Consulted and informed*: children are extensively consulted on a project
   designed and run by adults. One example is that of a New York
   television company which shows new programme ideas to a panel of
   children, has several pilot versions judged by them and subsequently
   redesigned. Other examples are those of surveys held among young
   people in various Canadian, American and Dutch cities to obtain their
   views on the renewal of their city and neighbourhoods, though not
   actually involving them in the analysis and the possible policy decisions.

6 *Adult-initiated, shared decisions with children*: in the case of projects
   concerned with community development, initiators such as policy-
   makers, community workers and local residents frequently involve
   various interest groups and age groups. An example of such projects in
   which children participate on an equal footing is the 'Nuestro Parque'
   project in East Harlem. Young children, teenagers and parents helped
   design a neighbourhood park, holding a display of their models for all

the residents, and after a round of consultation with everyone involved the plan was realized.

7 *Child-initiated and directed*: Children conceive, organize and direct a project themselves, without adult interference. Except in play, examples of this are hard to find, says the author, for the very reason that adults have difficulty in honouring children's initiatives and then leaving them to manage these themselves.

8 *Child-initiated, shared decisions with adults*: Hart considers this to be the highest rung on the ladder of participation, since he sees influence shared between children and adults as the final goal of participation. Students at a New York City high school formed a coalition for better sex education in schools, because they were concerned about the growing number of fellow students leaving the school on account of pregnancy. Having convinced the authorities by means of a petition of the value of their plans, peer counsellors were engaged by the schools to offer information, counselling and referral services on pregnancy and venereal diseases.

Participation projects in development countries

In the last few years children's participation has been increasingly considered as an instrument that can also improve the position of children 'in especially difficult circumstances'[8], notably in developing countries. This particularly applies to projects with street children in Asia, Latin America and Africa. So far, many governments consider confinement in prisons or other institutions the only remedy to keep these 'depraved and immoral young people' off the streets; or they turn a blind eye to the children being hunted, threatened and attacked by police, army or death squads[9]. The social image of these children as deviant, criminal and parasitic, says Panicker (involved in work with street children in India) is exactly what keeps them imprisoned in a system that solely recognizes disciplining as a solution (Panicker, 1989). Not only disciplining and repression, but also problematization proves to stand in the way of improvement in the situation of street children. During a conference about their situation held in April 1989, it was put forward that the way in which

[8]UNICEF uses this term to denote children without any family or who are so traumatized by disaster, poverty, wars, etc. that their basic needs cannot be met.

[9]This is reported upon with great regularity by Defence for Children International in the magazine *International children's rights monitor*.

this group of children is depicted in the media ('wretched, great poverty, awful misery' and usually very much romanticized) contributes little to an effective approach to the problems and quality of social work (see Ferrier & Clarijs, 1989). Several authors specifically censure the role of non-governmental organizations that invest a lot of money in small scale projects, reaching only a very small proportion of the children concerned. In this context these NGOs are engaged in fierce competition for the favour of their donor organizations. In order to survive, they are obliged to prove continually that they have sufficient 'clients' who appeal to the imagination; this means that children are not always being given a motivation and aid to restore contact with their relatives (Ferrier & Clarijs, 1989; Panicker, 1989, page 20).

The Brazilian professor Penna Firme (1989) argues in favour of replacing the view of street children as 'damaged individuals' by one in which they are seen as a subject of their own history and that of their people, and as having a lot of potential for the future: 'it is important to ask them what they know, what they have to give and what they can do' (ibid., page 30). Panicker is in favour of a similar perspective. She believes street children should be seen as they are: 'that is to say as hard-working, useful members of our society and as exploited, oppressed children who by their cheap labour in fact subsidize the cost of living of townspeople' (1989, page 19). She looks upon participation as an effective way to improve their situation. In the Butterflies Project, of which she is the director, the Bal Sabhas (a council of all children involved) decides what activities are undertaken. In this way the food supply, housing, education and health care have been organized cooperatively by the children. The foundation of such participation projects is usually laid by street workers (street educators and animators) who try to gain the confidence of small groups. They then cooperate with these groups in studying and charting their living conditions and the specific difficulties they have to deal with. A process of looking for solutions together has started. This sharing is a source of a possible strengthening of the children's position, because generally they try to survive purely individually. Indeed, their situation often causes fighting amongst themselves and competition. The choice of activities is emphatically left to the children themselves, the street workers having a facilitating role. They put forward various possibilities, help open doors to authorities and agencies, and assist in negotiation. Much attention is given to the organization of the groups themselves, notably in the form of developing democratic leadership. This approach has a twofold effect. In the first place the children's self-assurance, competence and solidarity are greatly stimulated, because they have come to belong to a mutual interest group. This strengthens their feeling of security, and lessens their (accurate) feeling of being entirely at the mercy of others. In the second place they discover that their actions can lead to tangible results. In a children's project for collecting scrap metal, paper etc. in Nairobi (Kenya) the children appeared to get a very raw deal from the middlemen who bought their wares. One reason was that the children were unable to read the scales, so that they were almost always cheated. Another was that as each individual child was so dependent on the merchants none of them ever dared to protest for fear of being excluded. The first activity the children asked the social worker concerned to undertake was a training in reading the scales and calculating prices on the basis of weight. Subsequently they developed a common strategy to become less dependent on the middlemen. They started selling the collected materials collectively to a factory which offered them a fixed price in exchange for a stable supply (Hart, 1992, page 30).

The objection that can justly be made against such projects is that they have little effect on the structural causes of the street children's problems. It is the fundamental lack of interest of authorities for these children that remains responsible, by the same mechanism as the economic exploitation of the Third World by the affluent West, for the deep poverty which is the very cause of the children being outcasts. Nevertheless this approach offers children some chance to survive in this type of hopeless situation, to recover their self-esteem and to develop a perspective on the future. Sometimes the projects even result in a political movement. In Brazil local groups of street children formed a national organization which has by now held a number of large conferences. These conferences received so much attention in the press that authorities were more or less forced to take action. In any case, street children in Brazil, thanks to organizing themselves, have achieved a voice of their own which it seems will actually benefit their living conditions (Penna Firme, 1989, page 32).

Conclusions

The UN Convention on the Rights of the Child has established, for the first time in history, that children's participation in society is among the fundamental human rights. After a great number of years in which attention was given mainly to protection and care – however badly these failed and still fail innumerable children – the freedom rights have now been defined. They are the basis for the recognition that children too are citizens, and may claim active involvement in matters concerning themselves and their living environment. In this chapter we have come to the conclusion that the way in which, and the extent to which, this happens are greatly dependent on the socio-cultural and political context in which these children live. In other words: children's participation is not a panacea or moral claim that is unvaryingly applicable in any situation. From the different definitions and differentiations reviewed it has appeared that participation:

- is a serviceable means of integrating young people into a given social structure without enabling them to exert any influence themselves *(fitting in)*

- may be a way to strengthen the social influence and power of young people *(empowerment)*

- may be instrumental in giving young people a chance to develop into competent, independent and responsible fellow citizens *(education in democratic citizenship)*.

It will be clear that 'fitting in' cannot be considered an active form of children's participation. Neither the development of young people nor that of society is served, because really this is just marking time: it does not effect any change, at best bringing the young into line. The validity of a perspective exclusively aimed at empowerment is very limited within the socio-cultural context of democratic welfare states. In contrast to the reality, in many parts of the world in which young people are literally exploited and abused, there seems to be hardly any question of organized repression in most western countries. Although there is room for improvement in the legal position of young people there as well, it is hard to maintain in general that they are entirely at the mercy of high-handed adults and authorities. Another argument against such one-sided accentuation of the power aspect is that in fact the importance of education, as well as of development of children, is then disregarded. We shall come back to this at greater length in the following chapters, but it may now be said that the power of young people should always be considered in relation to their current stage of development. Children fantasize about power, youngsters experiment with it. In both cases it is the task of parents and other educators to provide space for this, but also to set limits. This interaction is of outstanding importance to the social, cognitive and emotional development. It is also a reason why young people's desire of or need for power is difficult to make absolute. If, however, children are in a situation that does not meet primary conditions for existence (as is the case with street children in a number of developing countries), empowerment is of course a prerequisite. However, here too, education in citizenship appears to play a major part.

In line with the modern ideals of citizenship described in this chapter, children's and youth participation should comprise elements of education and influence. Participation as an educational instrument can be satisfactory only if young persons can derive true influence from it. Should this not be the case, they learn that democracy exists only in abstract. Conversely, participation as a means of strengthening children's power does not do sufficient justice to the importance of education and development. In modern western welfare states a type of intervention is needed which liberates less from oppression than from the web of problematization. Participation is not so much a remedy for repression as for depression. This means it is not only strengthening the formal power of young people that is at stake; taking them seriously and respecting their qualities should certainly concern us equally. Granting young people more influence is a major aspect of this, but it should not become an end in itself. If children are actively committed to community development, this will yield them more power. But they gain an equally important learning experience: we count, we are taken seriously, our ideas are appreciated, our environment evidently also belongs to us and therefore it is worth making an effort for. In other words: participation by children and young people is a way of enlarging the influence of the young on their own living situation and living environment, but it is also a way of shaping and strengthening their commitment to society. However, this educational perspective should not be idealized, i.e. formulated as an ideal standing apart from the material circumstances of children's lives and their expectations of the future. Such commitment can after all only develop when young people have an expectation of active support, from the society in which they grow up, for the realization of their fundamental claims as future citizens: a sound legal status, adequate scope for development and satisfying career prospects.

In this sense, the creation of possibilities for fellow citizenship and participation is the complete opposite of the presumption that youth is to be seen as a problem. The problem approach after all implies accentuation of everything that goes wrong or may go wrong with young people. Those who remain clear of such difficulties are in fact of no interest policy-wise, or to politics and to professionals. The reverse is the case where participating citizenship of young people is concerned: young people's potential and abilities are called upon, as well as their value for the future of (their) society. It is interesting in itself, but a derivative of this fundamental principle, that such an approach may also have preventive effects (cf. page 36)[10]. Stressing the positive forces in young people has both existential (personal) and social value. The life of young people becomes more meaningful, more challenging, and thus for many more joyful. In a socio-cultural context the platitude that youth has the future then loses its non-committal emptiness. Something can be done about it!

References

Arnstein S (1969) A ladder of citizen participation. *Journal of The American Institute of Planners*, July.

---

[10]This theme is worked out further in Chapters 3 and 6.

Castenmiller P (1989) Politieke participatie en politieke vorming. In: I Hartman & H Vlug (red) *Tussen burgerschap en eigenbelang. Participatie, legitimiteit en politieke vorming in de jaren '90.* Amsterdam/Leiden: Nederlands Centrum voor Democratische Burgerschapsvorming e.a. pp. 61–78.

Cohen S (1972) *Folk devils and moral panics. The creation of the Mods and the Rockers.* London: Martin Robertson.

Council of Europe (1993) *The development of an integrated approach to youth policy planning at local level.* Strasbourg: European Steering Committee for Intergovernmental Co-Operaration in the Youth Field (CDEJ).

Dahrendorf R (1988) *Burgerschap: het nieuwe vraagstuk.* Tekst Van der Leeuwlezing, Groningen 4-11-1988. Uitgave De Volkskrant: Amsterdam.

Ferrier J & R Clarijs (1989) Straatkinderen, zwerfjongeren. *Tijdschrift voor Jeugdhulpverlening en Jeugdwerk (TJJ),* jrg. 1, nr. 5–6. pp. 13–15.

Freire P (1972) *Pedagogie van de onderdrukten.* Baarn: Anthos.

Gunsteren HR van ea (1992) *Eigentijds burgerschap.* Rapport van de Wetenschappelijke Raad voor het Regeringsbeleid. 's-Gravenhage: SDU.

Hart RA (1992) *Children's participation. From tokenism to citizenship.* Florence, UNICEF Innocenti Essays nr. 4.

Hartman I (1989) De spanning tussen burgerschap en eigenbelang. Vijfentwintig jaar politiek vormingswerk in Nederland. In: I Hartman & H Vlug (red) *Tussen burgerschap en eigenbelang. Participatie, legitimiteit en politieke vorming in de jaren '90.* Amsterdam/Leiden: Nederlands Centrum voor Democratische Burgerschapsvorming e.a. pp. 15–34.

Kooy E van der (1989) Politieke vorming en marginalisering: Aufforderung zum Tanz? In: I Hartman & H. Vlug (red) *Tussen burgerschap en eigenbelang. Participatie, legitimiteit en politieke vorming in de jaren '90.* Amsterdam/Leiden: Nederlands Centrum voor Democratische Burgerschapsvorming ea pp. 167–76.

Langen M de (1991a) Recht voor kinderen. *Ars Aequi,* 40. pp. 213–21.

Langen M de (1991b) Kinderombudswerk. *Jeugd en Samenleving,* jrg. 21, nr. 12. pp. 770–7.

Linden FJ van der (1990) *Groot worden in een klein land. Feiten en cijfers uit het onderzoek naar de leefwereld van jongeren tussen 12 en 21 jaar.* Nijmegen: ITS.

Ling L (1993) *Internationale regelgeving over de rechten van het kind. Het VN-kinderrechtenverdrag vergeleken met andere mensenrechtendocumenten.* Amsterdam: Defence for Children International, afdeling Nederland.

Meeus W (1993) Jeugd en jeugdonderzoek in Nederland. De betekenis van 'Jongeren op de drempel van de jaren negentig' en 'Jeugd in Ontwikkeling' voor de kennis over de jeugd. *Jeugd en Samenleving*, 6/7. pp. 330–41.

Ministerie van Welzijn, Volksgezondheid en Cultuur (1991) *Samenwerken langs nieuwe wegen*. 's-Gravenhage: WVC-publicaties.

Ministerie van Welzijn, Volksgezondheid en Cultuur (1992) *Opvoedingssteun op maat. Hoofdlijnen pedagogische preventie in het kader van het jeugdbeleid*. 's-Gravenhage: SDU.

Ministerie van Welzijn, Volksgezondheid en Cultuur (1993a) *Jeugd verdient de toekomst. Nota intersectoraal jeugdbeleid*. 's-Gravenhage: WVC.

Ministerie van Welzijn, Volksgezondheid en Cultuur (1993b) *Jeugd betrekken. Een notitie over jeugdparticipatie*. Bijlage bij 'Jeugd verdient de Toekomst. Nota intersectoraal jeugdbeleid'. 's-Gravenhage: WVC.

Mollenhauer K (1986) *Vergeten samenhang. Over cultuur en opvoeding*. Meppel: Boom.

Nijnatten CHC van (red) (1993) *Kinderrechten in discussie*. Meppel: Boom.

Onvlee M (1992) Bespreking van 'Children without childhood' en een rapport van Amnesty International over de rechten van kinderen in Guatemala. *Tijdschrift voor de Rechten van het Kind*, nr. 2. pp. 11–12.

Panicker R (1989) Straatkinderen in India. *Tijdschrift voor Jeugdhulpverlening en Jeugdwerk (TJJ)*, jrg. 1, nr. 5–6. pp. 16–22.

Parlevliet C & S Sevenhuijsen (1992) *Zorg bekeken door een andere bril. Vrouwen en het debat over 'keuzen in de zorg'*. Utrecht: Metis.

Peeters J & C Woldringh (1993) *Leefsituatie van kinderen tot 12 jaar in Nederland*. Nijmegen: ITS.

Penna Firme T (1989) Straatkinderen in Brazilië. *Tijdschrift voor Jeugdhulpverlening en Jeugdwerk (TJJ)*, jrg. 1, nr. 5–6. pp. 29–35.

Raad voor het Jeugdbeleid (1991) *Meisjes en sociaal–culturele zelfstandigheid*. Amsterdam: Raad voor het Jeugdbeleid.

Raad voor het Jeugdbeleid (1992) *Zin in school. Een leefbare school voor een geschakeerde jeugd*. Amsterdam: Raad voor het Jeugdbeleid.

Sevenhuijsen S (1993) Feministische ethiek en de rechten van kinderen. In: CHC van Nijnatten (red) *Kinderrechten in discussie*. Meppel: Boom.

Veerman PE (1992) *The rights of the child and the changing image of childhood*. International Studies in Human Rights, Vol. 18. Dordrecht: Martinus Nijhof Publishers.

Voortman W (1991) *Participatie in jeugdbeleid. Inhoudsanalyse van het begrip participatie van jongeren in overheidsbeleid tussen 1945 en 1990*. Amsterdam: Vrije Universiteit, skriptie faculteit Pedagogische en Psychologische Wetenschappen.

Willis P (1990) *Common culture*. Boulder: Westview Press.

Winter M de (1986) *Het voorspelbare kind. VTO (vroegtijdige onderkenning van ontwikkelingsstoornissen) in wetenschappelijk en sociaal-historisch perspectief*. Lisse: Swets & Zeitlinger. Dissertatie Katholieke Universiteit Brabant.

Young IM (1992) *Equality, empowerment and social services. Some questions and problems*. Lezing NIZW, Utrecht, October 1992. (interne publicatie.)

Participation, upbringing and development

Introduction

So far, participation has been presented in contrast with a social approach that emphasizes the problems of children and young people, and as a means of contributing to the democratic development of citizenship. In this chapter, participation is looked at from the perspective of upbringing and development. Effecting active commitment to, and greater responsibility for, the living environment of the child, by the child, requires not only socio-political change, for example new forms of youth policy and strengthening of the socio-legal position of children, but also a thorough review of the way in which educators and children relate to each other, and of current attitudes towards the developmental process and the way in which this is influenced. The educational theories of this century encompass a number of movements in which the education of children and the development of society are considered as being closely related to each other. This is expressed in theoretical notions about, for example, education for citizenship, or for constructive participation in society, but also in concrete educational programmes which explore methods for community education. In such programmes, most of which were formulated by social educationalists, the participation of young people, although it may not have been referred to as such, played an important part. In the field of developmental psychology, direct references to active commitment and participation are noticeably less frequent. Since its conception, this discipline has focused particularly on understanding individual developmental processes and in doing so has constantly striven to attain the ideal of non-normative values. This is why participation as a normative goal of development or education is not an explicit subject of research or theorizing. However, developmental psychology does provide relevant knowledge about some of the conditions that may be considered essential to children's participation, in fields including cognitive, social and moral development. Moreover, this discipline provides an understanding of the way in which the active commitment of children influences the developmental process itself.

First of all we will look at the theoretical arguments and concrete initiatives that have been taken in the field of pedagogy to promote the active commitment and participation of children. Subsequently, we discuss some of the views of developmental psychologists. Finally, we consider the role of children's participation in the practical situation of raising children in the family. Although we have opted for a historical approach in this chapter by screening the two disciplines for concepts and interventions that seem relevant to children's participation, we do not claim to give a full historical overview. Our main aim is to look at the theories, experiments and research data that seem relevant to this subject.

The run-up to participation in history

All kinds of concepts and practices with respect to children, that today we consider to be perfectly normal, did not begin to play a part in history until children came to be seen as a special category of human beings. That is, from the time that the concept of youth started to mean something different to simply 'being young' in a world that does not give people special status or treatment on the grounds of age. *Upbringing* is the most striking example of this. This concept did not acquire its modern meaning of guidance to independence until this independence began to be postponed further and further. According to Dasberg (1975), education in this sense was virtually unknown in West-European culture until the eighteenth century. Children were looked after, protected and nourished until the age of six or seven, but after that they were regarded as 'pocket-sized adults' who, mostly out of sheer necessity, were made to join the work force[1]. Halfway through the eighteenth century, this view and this way of treating children provoked criticism. 'Enlightenment' thinkers such as Locke, Rousseau and Goethe pleaded for an educational moratorium in which children were to be exempted from adult duties and responsibilities for a prolonged period of time. They published writings in which children were depicted as good and rational beings. The fact that they nevertheless often grew up to be depraved adults was, in their view, the result of negative influences exerted by the environment and not, as had until then been generally accepted in Christian thought, of original sin. The conclusion that the enlightened thinkers drew from this was that children needed to be protected from the evils of the adult world. They were to be given the opportunity, space and freedom to develop, free of care, into conscious, happy and harmonious people. Thus the idea of a 'pedagogical province' developed (later referred to as 'youthland') in which children could be raised, freed from the need to work, shielded from exploitation and from the immoral influences of the street. This education – making the child aware of its possibilities – was at odds with what until then had been the

---

[1] cf. the differences of opinion of Peeters (1975), Röling (1982) and Noordman & van Setten (1989), also mentioned in Chapter 1.

customary practice of adjustment, indoctrination and training. Neither the interests of the state, the community, nor the church were to have priority, but the happiness of the individual. The prevailing line of thought was 'the more harmonious, positive-thinking and rationally operating adults, the better the world'. This enlightened way of thinking was able to take root at a time in which the European middle classes were gradually taking over economic and political power from the nobility and clergy. The prosperity and influence that resulted facilitated the rapid spread of these concepts of education throughout bourgeois circles. It was not until approximately 150 years later that the Enlightenment became a reality for the children of the poor and less powerful sections of the population.

The 'youthland' that was created in this way had enormous consequences for the relationship between children and society. On the one hand, the movement resulted in the protection of children against social exploitation. On the other hand, it increasingly isolated children 'for their own good' from the world of adults. Thus, a new problem developed, namely that of socialization. How could children be taught the competencies and skills that they needed to fulfil their future roles in society if they were deliberately excluded from this society? Mollenhauer (1986) uses the concepts of 'presentation' and 'representation' to illustrate this dilemma. As the worlds of children and adults were pulled further apart, a process that, according to Mollenhauer, had already started in the fifteenth century, the direct presentation of adult ways of life to children was increasingly impeded. Because children were less directly involved in the day-to-day reality of their parents and the community, the possibilities for them to familiarize themselves with its content and structure through experience fell away. Instead of this, the educational genre of representation developed. Education was no longer a confrontation *with* reality, but a reflection *of* reality. One of the first and, at the same time, most influential examples of this genre is the work of Comenius entitled *Orbis sensualium pictus* that was published in 1658. It was, literally, the universe in pictures, a schematic arrangement of reality using pictures and symbols with which Comenius wanted to structure the complexity of the big world for children, it being for them both incomprehensible and inaccessible. According to Mollenhauer, this reflection in theatrical form serves as a model for modern education. Questions such as 'what should children learn?', 'how should the subject matter be taught?' and 'how can children be motivated to absorb this?' have their roots in the creation of a separate educational sphere.

As the institutionalization of youthland progressed – the period of youth became longer and longer, and the educational walls, literally and figuratively, higher and higher – cracks in the fortress became visible. These came from within and from without, that is to say, from the perception that children had or were assumed to have of their environment, and from society. As far as the first problem is concerned: Dasberg speaks of an 'increasingly traumatic period of puberty' resulting from the tension between maturity at an ever younger age, and emancipation at an ever later age (Dasberg, 1975, page 114). From the educational and psychological literature on puberty and adolescence that began to appear approximately 100 years ago, the picture does in fact emerge of a developmental phase accompanied by violent emotional tensions and conflicts. We deliberately use the word 'emerge' because the young people concerned virtually never expressed their views in such publications, and because the nature of the problems that were described would seem to be highly coloured by the norms and values held by most of the authors. At the end of the nineteenth century, says de Graaf, puberty was 'discovered', mainly by psychiatrists, as a dangerous period in a psychopathological sense, particularly with respect to sexual development and socially unacceptable behaviour such as criminality. A little later, following the publication of Stanley Hall's standard work on adolescence in 1904[2], the transitional phase between childhood and adulthood came to be seen as a 'normal problem' requiring the full attention of educationalists and psychologists. The conclusion was that during this phase the basis was laid for the development of the personality, for intellectual, emotional and social development, and for the social integration of young people: 'puberty became a new norm for psychic growth' (de Graaf, 1989, pages 111–114)[3]. At the same time, a second problem came to light. Not only had this phase of life been discovered as a major source of psychic problems and tension for young people themselves, it was also a source of danger for the social order. Puberty was seen as a period in which young people were likely to indulge in sexual excesses and criminality. It is in this light that the first arguments in favour of children's and youth participation were heard; at that time, of course, worded differently. Puberty theorists saw the self-rule of young people within the educational system as an important educational means of rationalizing the aimless and therefore 'dangerous' needs of puberty along constructive lines. The school councils and student councils that were founded during the 1920s in some American, British, German and Dutch schools can be seen in this light.

Participation and social education

The scientific pedagogy that was practised until the beginning of this century had been characterized since the Enlightenment by strong individualism. German philosophers such as Immanuel Kant and Friedrich

---

[2]Hall (1904).

[3]See also, for example: Bertels (1978 a,b).

Herbart saw 'moral perfection of the individual' and 'mastery over the self' as the most important aims of education. In his *Contrat social* and *Emile*, Rousseau expressed a comparable point of view. The idea that education should serve individual happiness and the full development of the personality meshed perfectly with the development of the bourgeois culture that had been taking place in the countries of Western Europe since the Enlightenment (cf. Chapter 1). In this view, the rational, free individual was seen as the motor of economic, social and cultural progress; knowledge and personal 'civilization' formed the key to the established bourgeois elite. Around 1900, a counter-movement, 'Sozialpädagogik', began to manifest itself within education, particularly in Germany. The traditional 'Individualpädagogik' was criticized because it saw human development as extremely divorced from society. 'Der Mensch wird zum Menschen allein durch menschliche Gemeinschaft', was the thesis of the philosopher Natorp (1899) who is regarded as the godfather of this movement (Coumou & van Stegeren, 1987). According to Natorp, ethical principles such as sincerity, justice and social courage developed through taking part in social life, and not merely in the seclusion of the relationship between educator and child. In his view, therefore, education is by definition a social matter: education and community cannot exist independently of one another. Natorp, and, for example, also Kerschensteiner (1917) expressed their views in educational reform or proposals for it. Both were opposed to the authoritarian, class-bound Prussian system of education which, in their view, preserved the enormous differences in social status between the young people from the various strata of society. Thus, around the turn of the century, Kerschensteiner founded an 'Arbeitsschule' in Munich, in which the individual initiatives and responsibility of young people played a central role. 'Community education' was the creed, an ideal that critics, however, were quick to interpret as an argument in favour of education by the state. In the Netherlands too, these ideas were received with scepticism. While influential educationalists such as Bavinck (1916) and Kohnstamm (1919) were in favour of education for community and citizenship, they were strongly opposed to a collectivist, Marxist interpretation of this. According to them, community education had in the first place to be given form within the individual educational learning situation. Learning to think independently, and to be accountable to oneself, was a condition for this (Vermeer, 1987; Carpay, 1994).

According to Mennicke (1937)[4], deliberate social-educational measures, aimed at social integration, had become a historical necessity because of the dismantling of traditional class society. This society, founded on 'self-care within relatively small circles' was both economically and psychologically

---

[4] Mennicke was a German educationalist who fled from the Nazi regime to the Netherlands in 1933.

'inevitable' for its members: 'the existence of the individual was only ensured if he integrated into the whole of a particular group, namely the class' (ibid., page 33). The lack of real alternatives (other than being ostracized) meant that there was no question of a social-educational problem. Within a traditionally organized community, educating and being educated was virtually synonymous with survival. According to Mennicke, the social-educational strength of class society decreased as more and more states were formed, civil freedom expanded, and thought became rationalized. From the second half of the nineteenth century onwards, this problem became more acute. Besides economic growth, industrialization also brought about widespread poverty that 'divorced people from their traditional circumstances and removed them to forms of habitation, working and living that deprived them of any kind of footing because all relations with the bonds of tradition had been broken'. This 'asocial-ness' resulted in social protest and 'attempts at revolution, in the face of which the social-educational resources of this century were totally inadequate' (ibid., pages 42–3). In this context of social unrest and resistance, the concept of community education was given a powerful boost. Of course, the way in which this was interpreted was strongly determined by politics and ideology. Mennicke distinguishes three variants. The first form is *reactive*: society feels threatened by youth and tries to fight the symptoms of this danger without realizing how these are interrelated with the developments in society itself. As an example of this, he mentions the fight against the phenomenon of criminal and neglected youth in the lower social classes by means of strict detention centres and 'internal mission' (religious influences). The Nursery School Movement described by Singer (1989) can also be seen in this light. The main aim of this kind of child care, that developed around the beginning of the nineteenth century on the initiative of liberal-minded citizens and enlightened aristocrats, was to 'protect' young children from poor homes against the unwholesome influences of the family, and to protect society against criminality, corruption and godlessness. As a second variant, Mennicke mentions the *conscious, free forms of education* (of which he himself was an adherent). This involves social-educational measures that are based on the realization that modern society requires an artificial supplement for the gaps that have been left in its power to educate. The most important areas in which these measures are to take effect are psychological–spiritual development and social experience. In this connection he sees an important task for the free youth movement, which can offer young people spiritual meaning and opportunities for 'gaining experience in society in the form of a free mutual struggle'. The latter was needed because (due to the technologizing and mechanizing of labour) the experiences gained in free collaboration, and also the opportunity to exercise social skills day by day, in a natural way, had largely been lost. The third variant is the *conscious, but compulsive form of education*. By this Mennicke refers to the social-educational interventions of the two major totalitarian systems that characterized his time: communism and Nazism. In both cases, it is the state that takes over education. The total, rationalized state regards the family as basically unreliable, and tries to consolidate its grip on all socializing agencies. Where, in the case of the second variant, the issue is to intensify 'the free-working educational strength of society in such a way that each member of that society comes to free inner acceptance of the whole', the 'organizational strength of totalitarian education is so all-embracing that nothing is left to the spontaneity of individuals' (Mennicke, 1937, pages 85–94).

Community education thus appears to be a concept that fits many theories. For it is the way in which community is defined that determines what the aims of education are to be. When this is seen as a collection of free, independent individuals, then community education and Individual-pädagogik are virtually in line with one another[5,6]. If, on the other hand, we argue not from a personal, but from a collective ideal of equality, then community education takes on the character of a (voluntary or involuntary) integration strategy. Despite these fundamental differences, there does appear to be a certain convergence when it comes to choosing educational methods. Thus, famous educationalists such as Makarenko and Korczak have experimented with various forms of self-government by children on the basis of totally divergent educational points of view. Makarenko did this with neglected and vagrant children in two Ukrainian communes in the period between 1920 and 1935. Group responsibility carried to an extreme was seen to be subservient to the dominant collectivist ideology (cf. Goodman, 1949). During the 1930s, in his home for Jewish orphans in Warsaw, Janusz Korczak (1920) developed the children's court, the children's parliament and the children's newspaper as components of a

---

[5]Mennicke argues that Rousseau's educational theories can definitely also be characterized as a form of community education. Placed in the perspective of his time, in which 'the great inequality between people, and groups of people, that had resulted from the unrestrained use of power and deception by the clergy, brought about tensions that made community education impossible', individualistic education was intended to 'give everyone equal conditions for their development by having everyone grow up, as far as possible, under the same influences'. The fact that it was precisely this community element that failed in the social–educational programme of the Enlightenment, according to Mennicke, is because it was inconsistent with the historical reality: 'the disrupting force of rationalism was greater than its constructive possibilities' (Mennicke, 1937, p. 23–4).

[6]Owen's educational experiment (around 1824) in England with group education of young children outside the family, is an elaboration of the Enlightenment ideal that was also inspired by ideas of community education. According to Owen, it was the family that stood in the way of community feeling, and this is why, in his New Lanark Infant School, he tried to teach children that their personal happiness and the happiness of the community were interdependent. 'Learning to be reasonable in the face of reality' was the key concept in his thinking about moral and intellectual education' (from Singer, 1989, p. 92).

form of education based on equality and mutual respect between children and adults. And around 1920, on the basis of a radical–liberal philosophy, A.S. Neill founded 'Summerhill' in England, a school that wanted to have done with oppression and obedience. The pupils enjoyed great freedom and governed the school according to democratic principles (Sommerville, 1982). In the Netherlands, the Werkplaats Kindergemeenschap (Workshop Children's Community) in Bilthoven, founded in 1926 by Kees Boeke and Beatrice Cadbury, was a striking example of educational reform in which the pupils (workers) played an important role in the decision-making of the school (cf. Kuipers, 1992).

Although we cannot draw conclusions about the actual spread of children's and youth participation during the first half of this century, we can state with some certainty that the idea occupied an important place in the educational debate. The main scene of action was found in the movements for mature youth. During the 1920s and 1930s, all kinds of youth organizations came into being on a political and/or religious basis, such as the Wandervögel, Scouts, and youth clubs. Selten (1991) calls the most striking characteristic of such movements the 'generation conscious-ness'. This manifested itself in an individual style and culture in which young people tried to express the ideal of 'being-young-together'[7]. The shaping of this ideal brought with it long discussions concerning the extent to which autonomy and self-government were part of the essence of the movement. Proponents considered active 'self-regulation' to be an important educational tool for community education (Eernstman, 1926, cit. Selten, page 13). Others repudiated this principle, precisely for educational reasons. The leadership of the Catholic youth movement, for example, was of the opinion that the autonomy of young people did not fit into the main goal of the movement: training for the 'evangelization of youth'. Our impression is that the majority of educationalists, although mostly fervent proponents of the youth movement, attached greater importance to the possibilities for psychological manipulation (youth idealism) than to social education through active participation. For that matter, de Rooy (1982) designates the youth movement as 'the culmination of youthland', precisely because of the very isolated position that it claimed with respect to the adult world (page 131).

After the Second World War, an identity crisis gradually precipitated within Dutch social education. Not only did it lose ground in the world of science to individually-oriented sub-disciplines such as remedial education and clinical pedagogy, but it got caught up in a theoretical debate about the

---

[7]A term used by van Hessen (1965). Apart from his work, the reader is referred, among others, to Harmsen (1961), de Rooy (1982), and Selten (1991) for further analyses and descriptions of the youth movements that arose in the Netherlands during this period.

content and place of the discipline itself. In the meantime, social-educational practice (including socio-cultural training and youth work) was losing its contact with young people; this type of work particularly failed to come to grips with unschooled factory workers (de Rooy, ibid., page 138). During the seventies, both the academic and applied branches of social education developed in a direction that was more and more critical of the social structure. Emphasis shifted to the (disadvantaged) social position of young people, and to the structures underlying this. Concepts such as 'public consultation', 'assertiveness' and 'emancipation' emerged: the discovery of youth as a critical potential for social change (Dibbits, 1987; Abma, 1993). However, it proved difficult to 'sell' such social-educational analyses to young people, particularly the disadvantaged. Obviously, the participation of young people cannot be proclaimed on the basis of the ideological propositions of adults. It seems that more insight is needed into the motives and the living environment of the young people themselves. Consequently, from the 1970s onwards, this has been the most important theme of social-educational research. Participation does not come back into the picture until the beginning of the 1990s when ways and means are sought to strengthen the involvement of youth in local youth policy within the framework of social reform (cf. Hazekamp *et al.*, 1993).

Children's participation and developmental psychology

Present-day developmental psychology presents itself mainly as a science that in an empirical descriptive way, is in search of patterns in the way children develop. In this sense, it is distinguished from pedagogy which regards itself as a normative science, and is engaged in the study of 'the extent to which the development of children can be influenced by a view of educationally desirable goals that is justified on the basis of normative science' (Miedema & van Ijzendoorn, 1992, page 262). Because of this emphasis, questions that involve value judgements such as 'what is good for a child?' and 'which educational and developmental goals are desirable for the community?' play a background role in developmental psychology. And therefore, the discipline raises the question of children's and youth participation as a goal of social education. Nevertheless, a developmental psychological approach is relevant for two reasons. Firstly, fundamental debates about the way in which developmental processes are to be considered have been going on within developmental psychology for a long time. The discussion itself is important in this context because the different points of view provide insight into the image of young people that is created in modern society, as well as society's attitude towards the young. Some people consider empirical-analytical developmental psychology to be anything but a neutral, value-free science, and blame the implicit views of this discipline for the relative isolation in which western youth finds itself in regard to the adult world (cf. Skolnick, 1976). Secondly, developmental psychology has come up with a number of insights indicating that insufficient scope for participation can be a restraining factor in the developmental process. Conversely, the active commitment of children to their social environment can be seen as an important condition for stimulating development and psychosocial well-being.

Views of development and society

What role do concepts such as participation, citizenship and social commitment play, explicitly or implicitly, in the thinking about children's development? In order to answer this question, we first briefly sketch the history of developmental psychology: how do various well-known theorists describe the relations between the individual development of children and the development of society? In practical terms, after all, whether one takes, for example, a maturation hypothesis (development as a biologically controlled process) as the point of departure for raising and educating children, or an hypothesis (development as the result of social influences) can make a great difference. Strictly speaking, in the case of the first view, there is little about the socialization process that can be controlled, because the course of development is largely determined by the constitution. From the point of view of the second hypothesis, control is all the more important because development is actually little else than the result of the socialization process. And it is precisely this that raises the question of what the goal of childhood development is, or to put it differently, how and in what direction this process should be influenced.

The idea that the development of children could be an interesting object of scientific study arose, just as was the case with education, during the Enlightenment. Influential educationalists such as Comenius, Locke and Rousseau based their educational counsels on observations and descriptions of children, from which development emerged as a natural process. According to these authors, this process could, with a great deal of patience and guidance, be transformed along rational lines by educators. During the same period, various children's biographies were written, among others by the Swiss educationalist Pestalozzi (in 1774) and his German contemporary Tiedeman (in 1787). It can justly be said of these that they contain developmental psychological ideas which were ahead of their time (cf. Dennis, 1972). However, the origin of 'real' developmental psychology is not attributed to these authors because their work is usually labelled as subjective and prescriptive. Generally, therefore, the publication of

Darwin's *Origin of species* in 1859 is designated the starting point. This book laid the foundation for evolutionary thought about children. Development is conceptualized as a biological process which unfolds from the individual. Inspired by these views, the so-called 'Child Study Movement' arose several decades later in the United States and Europe. This movement of scientists, led by Stanley Hall, urged that such evolutionary insights be put into practice in upbringing and education. In Hall's publications, the so-called recapitulation theory played an important role. Childhood development (ontogenesis) was seen as an accelerated recurrence of the development of the human species as a whole (phylogenesis). Hall saw the traits and characteristics of children as being determined by heredity, and from that he concluded that education should obey the laws of nature. He believed that education had little effect on the child until puberty. According to Hall, parents did best to limit themselves to regulating and disciplining the child until that time (Hall, 1904). Quite at odds with these views were the progressive concepts of Hall's contemporary and fellow-countryman, John Dewey. The latter based his educational ideas on what he called an instrumentalist developmental concept: children develop not only according to abstract natural laws, but especially through confrontation with elements in the social context with which they would also be confronted as adults. We mention Dewey's work here, not so much because it was very influential within the field of developmental psychology, but because he can be seen as an American representative of 'community education' (cf. page 51). His developmental concept resulted in a form of education which, in the first instance, was aimed at democratizing society. Learning to work together on activities that are socially meaningful for children was an essential component (see page 114).

During the first decades of this century, the image of developmental psychology was determined by the nature–nurture debate: is the development of a child determined by its predisposition or by the environment? Hall, and later Gesell (1928), were the most important representatives of the first view. Gesell saw development as a maturation process that passes through a number of fixed stages. The environment plays a marginal role in this: at most, it can accelerate or delay the transition to the next stage of development. The most important task of educators was to adapt themselves to the 'intrinsic' growth rate and the possibilities of the child. Behaviourists like Thorndike, Watson and Skinner, on the other hand, were of the opinion that development is nothing more than a cumulative learning process. Behaviour, emotions and intelligence were to be regarded as the results of conditioning which could be totally controlled by the parents. In their view, raising children was in fact a form of behaviour modification. This point of view created not only educational expectations but also socio-political ones. Thorndike (1913), for example, believed that the human species could be improved by means of 'social engineering': the systematic and controlled application of learning principles on a large scale. Watson

(1925) saw in the mystique of innate differences the most important obstacle to social freedom and equality. By means of proper guidance (read: conditioning) every healthy child could be trained for any and every occupation (page 91), regardless of his talents, his special circumstances, or his descent. Psychological support for the ideology of the American Dream! This optimism about the extent to which man and society could be shaped by government policy was, at the same time, a notable reason why psychoanalytical theorizing, after an initially warm welcome in circles of the Child Study Movement, for a long time played a marginal role in the evolution of developmental psychological theory (Ingleby & Goudena, 1992, page 172). Freud's position with respect to the inevitable, discordant and irrational nature of the early development of the child was rejected by the behaviourists as pessimistic and speculative (ibid.).

In Europe, psychologists such as Piaget and Vygotsky tried, each in his own way, to break away from what they saw as a too strongly accentuated dichotomy between nature and nurture. Piaget studied the development of cognitive structures in children, and formulated a theory characterizing development as a process of phases in which the child, via internal mechanisms such as assimilation and adaptation, learns to understand his environment better (cf. Piaget, 1923, 1963). According to him, the structure of mental development is a biological fact. While it is true that learning (by way of upbringing and education) can influence the content of thought, it does not influence the cognitive structures themselves (Elbers, 1988, page 3). The Soviet psychologist Vygotsky (1929) adopted quite a different view of the relationship between development and learning. He states that cognitive development can only occur through 'learning processes that stimulate development'. With guidance from adults, children learn to go beyond the possibilities of their own cognitive development at that particular time (the actual level of development). Vygotsky called the level that the child is able to reach with the help of adults, but not yet able to reach on his own, the 'zone of nearest development'. Contrary to Piaget's view, education has to precede development. In this, the adult is 'the embodiment of the culture into which the child grows. The adult who associates with the child conveys the historical achievements of human society to the child' (van Parreren, 1979, page 199).

With the movements described thus far we have also outlined the context within which post-war developmental psychology evolved, a context in which the nature–nurture debate continued. However, it did lose a lot of its edge with the rise of so-called interactionist approaches, in which both the role of disposition and that of the environment were recognized (cf. Sameroff, 1975). Empirical-analytical research, inspired particularly by behaviourism, now dominated the discipline. This resulted in an ever more microscopic study of human development. On the one hand, there was thematic fragmentation (into functional, cognitive, social, and personality development, etc.), on the other hand the developmental process increasingly came to be seen as independent of its social and cultural context. Kessen (1983) typified the childhood image of modern developmental psychology as 'individual' and 'self-contained'. According to him, this picture is a reflection of the dominant values and standards of researchers and society, rather than something that can be taken as being universal. Historical and cross-cultural comparison show that the developmental profile of children is largely dependent on 'major forces in culture', such as the enormous social regard for science and technology in our own time (page 30). From the 1970s onward, this kind of comment on the asocial, acultural and ahistorical character of developmental psychology has been expressed by a very mixed company of scientists, from different disciplines and inspired by different forms of social and scientific criticism (for a review see: Ingleby, 1986). Bronfenbrenner (1979a), for example, argues in favour of 'ecological' developmental research, in which children would no longer be studied exclusively in alienating test or laboratory situations, but in their own day-to-day living environment. This means a considerable broadening of the field that should be studied by developmental psychologists. According to Bronfenbrenner, the ecological environment in which development occurs, consists of four levels, namely the *micro-system* (the complex of relations between the individual and environment), the *meso-system* (the relations between the different environments in which the individual finds himself), the *exo-system* (the formal and informal social structures in the direct environment, such as the neighbourhood, school, etc.), and finally, the *macro-system* (general structures such as the dominant cultural, social, educational, legal and political systems, of which the micro-, meso-, and exo-systems are concrete manifestations). Developmental psychology that studies individual characteristics and that regards these environmental influences as more or less constant, maintains above all the status quo: 'to the extent that we take environments into account in our study, we select and treat them more or less as sociological constants rather than as evolving social systems that are open to interesting new transformations' (Bronfenbrenner, 1979b, page 421).

This last point is an important observation if we want to consider the subject of children's and youth participation from the perspective of developmental psychology. After all, the study and theorizing within this field have for a long time focused on the description, analysis and explanation of the actual development within the existing social context. In so far as there is any experimenting with environmental influences in a study, these usually consist of the manipulation of a few variables in the micro-system. As we have seen, the possibilities for social participation in the present social world by children and young people are very limited. This is partly the result of the concept of development in which individual development is isolated from its ecological environment (cf. 'the individual and self-contained child'). According to Bronfenbrenner, this concept changes when 'research into the ecology of human development also includes experiments that involve innovative restructuring of prevalent ecological systems, in ways that deviate from existing institutional ideologies and structures by redefining aims, roles and activities and by introducing connections between systems that previously existed in isolation of each other' (1979b, page 421). However, as far as present knowledge about the relationship between development and participation is concerned, we have to make do with insights that were gained in a context that usually did not extend beyond the individual child's brain, or the interaction between educator and child. Although the social involvement and social responsibility of children is formulated now and again as a far-off developmental objective, systematic research into and theorizing about the preconditions that lead to such objectives have thus far been virtually lacking.

Development and participation

Taking these limitations into consideration, what can we now say about children's and youth participation from the point of view of developmental psychology? First of all, we look at modern notions of early child development. A lot of theorists are of the opinion that the quality of social interaction between young children and their parents is of overriding importance for the further course of (social) development (cf. Bremner, 1987). During the last decades, there have been important shifts in the ideas about the course of this process. Young children who, for a very long time, were seen as passive, helpless and self-centred beings, are gradually being 'discovered' as competent, influential participants in the process of their own social and mental development. Both researchers who emphasize the biological origin of human behaviour, and researchers who stress the role of the social environment seem to have come to the conclusion that children, from a very early age, are constantly working to actively shape their relationship with the social world. Many studies that were carried out after the 1950s and 1960s and which, among others, found expression in a book entitled *The competent infant* (Stone et al., 1973), contradict what until then had been the dominating concept of the young child as a passive partner in a symbiotic duality with its mother. In particular, Bowlby's study on bonding processes drew attention to the existence of social signalling systems with which the young child can initiate the process, such as crying, smiling, and affectionate behaviour (van Ijzendoorn, 1985). According to Bowlby, the quality of the bonding is determined particularly by the sensitivity with which the primary carer reacts to the signals of the baby. If this process inspires a sense of safety and confidence in the child, it develops an internal theory ('working model') which enables it to cope with later social and emotional relations in a positive way. In *The psychological birth of the human infant,* the child analyst Margaret Mahler describes how, after an 'autistic phase' of several months, babies become more and more oriented to the outside world. In this way, on the one hand the process of individuation is started, and on the other hand the primary symbiotic relationship with the mother is weakened. She considers both aspects to be of great importance for the development of the sense of self. Now, according to Mahler, young children by nature vary greatly in the extent to which they structure this process: active babies are inclined to mobilize their entire behavioural repertoire in response to a light stimulus, and are very actively oriented to their environment, while less active babies tend mainly to look around, and are better able to comfort themselves (orally) (Mahler, 1975, 1983).

Researchers such as Emde (1983) and Stern (1983) have emphasized the interactive nature of this early development of the personality. Both assume a biologically based mutual reward mechanism between the parent and child, in which the caring behaviour of the parent is closely related to the emotional and social utterances of the child. According to these researchers, the sensitivity with which the parent reacts to the ever more differentiated signals of the child, is of overriding importance to the later social and emotional functioning of the child. Children who in their early childhood have learned that affectivity is used manipulatively by adults, are more likely themselves to learn to manipulate rather than empathize. Conversely, when they are never confronted with the manipulative use of affect, this could result in 'social naivety' (Stern, ibid.). Developmental psychologists such as Bruner (1977) and Kaye (1982) were opposed to the biological determinism that was the basis for the ideas of the above-mentioned researchers. Their studies on the early development of children emphasize the social construction process of the personality and of sociability, in the tradition of Vygotsky. This view also ascribes to young children significant capabilities for communicating and for controlling social interaction, but here the task of educators extends beyond responding with empathy to the signals of the child. Parents continually interpret the behaviour of their child and thus give it meaning. In fact, according to these researchers, they fulfil the role of a teacher, because by offering the child ever more complex tasks, they stimulate the child to more mature patterns of social interaction. If this 'dialogue' and 'joint action' is well-structured and stimulated by the parents, the child gets to know itself and the world, and is in a position to internalize the conventions and rules of the culture.

According to Piaget (1923, 1955), the process in which the child develops from an 'egocentric' being to a socially communicative person, is mainly intellectual in character. For babies, apart from primary care, interaction with carers is of little importance, because their cognitive structure does not yet make them capable of distinguishing between themselves and others. In Piaget's view, the social use of language does not become possible until somewhere between the fourth and seventh year. Not until after that can communicative thought begin to develop. Piaget and his followers, however, were criticized for having neglected the social character of the cognitive development process. Elbers (1988), for example, argues that the ideas of children originate not only in the use of their own intellectual strategies, but also in the strategies that adults transfer to them. This means that the content of that adult knowledge, at the very least partly determines how children learn to interpret their environment. If parents pay little attention to the knowledge and motivation that is required for participation and social commitment, then children will probably not, or only much later, pick up this competence. Secondly, there is a lot of criticism on the age phasing that Piaget used. Although he himself often pointed out that it was a question of averages, various critical experiments have demonstrated that the age limits found were partly the result of the study methods used (cf. Elbers, ibid., pages 41–59). In their experiments, Vygotsky and his later colleagues, El'Konin and Davydov, demonstrated that 'education that stimulates development' could lead children to capabilities that according to Piaget were unlikely to occur in a particular phase. Thus it appeared to be possible to teach children of seven years and older to work with abstract concepts, with relations between concepts, and with the properties of these relations. Moreover, it appeared that children were capable of reflecting on their own activities at a much earlier age than Piaget had assumed (van Parreren, ibid., page 200). The British developmental psychologist Donaldson, is of the opinion that children have far greater social and cognitive potential than educators and schools often assume. In her book, *Children's minds* (1978), she claims that many inherent and acquired social and cognitive capabilities are insufficiently utilized because education confronts children with tasks whose purpose or meaning they do not always understand. In other words, they are asked to solve problems without being able to see the connection with their day-to-day reality, and without learning to understand the significance of the problems. As a result, many children do not become sufficiently aware of their own intellectual and social capabilities with the result that their sense of control over their own thinking and actions remains underdeveloped. According to Donaldson, children are kept dependent in many areas too long, as a result of which they are denied the possibility of gaining experience in 'their considerable capacity for individual initiative and responsible action' (ibid., page 113). All this means that a considerable number of children give up their basic human need to develop into effective, competent and independent people at an early age, and start to regard themselves as stupid and useless to society. Obviously, this can also affect the need for social participation or, in any case, weaken its development.

In the previous section, the development of children and young people was described as a process of mutual interaction (transactions) between the individual and his/her environment. In this context, Elbers, following

Valsiner, refers to a culturally determined field of development: 'the growing psychological properties of a child are a response to the physical, cultural and social circumstances, challenges and obstacles which it encounters' (Elbers, 1993, page 83; Valsiner, 1987). Thus the possibilities and limitations that the environment offers children, channel the developmental process. In recent years, various child and developmental psychologists have pointed out that many children find it difficult to fulfil some of the developmental tasks some people set them[8]; it is thought that their environment offers them too little room for learning and development. These researchers now see the expansion and facilitation of these possibilities as a measure that serves to prevent psychosocial problems and behaviour disorders. Participation thus becomes a means of realizing these developmental tasks (educational theorists would speak of 'educational objectives'). An example is the following developmental task in adolescence mentioned by Diekstra (1992): 'The development of an individual system of norms and values together with an ethical and political awareness, consistent with the behaviour and actions of the individual; so that in the long term responsible action is possible, both in private life and in public' (page 119). From a psychological point of view he considers the realization of such a task (education for citizenship) of great importance, particularly with respect to the *forming of an identity*, but also as a means of preventing problem behaviour such as criminality. Consequently, Diekstra argues in favour of preventive measures aimed at 'offering adolescents appropriate opportunities to express and present themselves, to be able to put thoughts and ideas into practice (ibid., page 150). According to this author, schools in particular should be 'targets' of intervention. He believes that schools have until now failed miserably because they generally make pupils adopt passive behaviour or behaviour that is lacking in initiative. He also considers it 'crucial that adolescents themselves be able to participate in the creation of their living and learning situation, so that they can identify in a more positive way with the social institutions with which they are confronted ... and so that feelings of alienation can be countered' (ibid., page 150).

Research into moral development also provides good psychological arguments for strengthening the active participation of children, also younger ones, in processes in the 'real' world. Analogous to the way in

---

[8]The concept of developmental tasks, introduced in 1972 by Havinghurst, is currently the cause of heated debate within the field of developmental psychology. This discussion mainly concerns the normative or non-normative character of this concept. Although the author is of the opinion that it is never possible to define developmental tasks without value judgements, if only because different cultures have different views of what is meant by 'desirable development' (cf. de Winter, 1986), such studies are mentioned because they give us insight into the empirical relationships between developmental processes and current social (thus normative) expectations.

which Piaget described the development of thought, Kohlberg sketches the development of a sense of values in children as the result of intellectual growth. In his theory he speaks of six universal stages of moral development that have a fixed sequence (Kohlberg, 1979). These stages represent, not so much the (culture-dependent) content of thought, but the reasoning process by which children reach moral judgements. Heymans (1992, page 163), on the other hand, argues that 'current moral development, as empirically encountered, is partly the result of cultural practices in which children and young people are not, or not always, taken as serious actors'. Thus styles of upbringing (both within and outside the family) in which power differences are stressed (the so-called authoritarian style) have an inhibiting effect on moral development. Participation (for example, doing household work) on the other hand, provides an important resource for that same moral development (Goodnow, 1988, cit. Heymans, ibid.). Consequently, he argues in favour of well-considered access to, and experience with, the working world of adults, which could be discussed in school (Heymans, ibid., page 191). The work of the American develop-mental psychologist Damon (1988), leads us to draw comparable conclusions. On the grounds of studies on cognitive, social and moral development, he concludes that morality is learned particularly through active participation in the 'natural context of tangible social interactions'. Thus he rejects the view that morality can be stimulated by means of the abstract procedures of clarifying values that have been much in use lately: 'For a child, the outcome of a social engagement – its developmental 'message' – is determined more by the quality and method of the child's participation than by ideas to which the child might be exposed' (page 146). For this reason, one of the things he advocates, as does Kohlberg (1985), is the transformation of schools into 'participatory democracies, in which pupils as well as teachers are responsible for drawing up and maintaining school rules and rules of behaviour' (cf. page 112).

Over the past years, a lot of research has been done into the way in which the thinking and reasoning of parents about upbringing, influences the *social-cognitive development* of children. In this area of development, the concept of 'seeing in perspective' plays an important role. Selman (1976) defines this as a developmental process in which 'individuals learn to understand the relationship between their own perspective and that of others'. For children's participation this would seem to be an essential precondition because, after all, democratic functioning at the very least assumes a measure of understanding for other points of view. Studies by Dekovic, Janssens and Gerris (1989) show that the level at which parents themselves are capable of 'seeing in perspective', strongly influences the cognitive development of their children. Parents raising their children who act on the basis of their own needs, or on the basis of conventional rules and norms, appear to relate quite differently to their children than do parents who take the position and needs of the child into account. The former are generally more restrictive (aiming for obedience), give less explanation about rules, and do little to stimulate the child to form its own opinion. Parents whose thought processes appear more 'child-oriented', are more likely to address the child's own sense of responsibility, and to urge it to see other people's points of view. According to the researchers, the development of social cognition in children is facilitated by this style of upbringing (ibid., page 211). Hart, finally, emphasizes the importance of children's participation for the development of *autonomy* and *social cooperation*. Because children are involved in 'real projects' they discover that dialogue and negotiation with other children and with adults is indispensable. This 'learning to work together' is in its turn a precondition for the development of autonomy (Hart, 1992, page 42).

The conclusion that must be drawn from such findings is that, in our culture, generally accepted developmental goals such as independence, responsibility, autonomy and employing perspective – which are necessary for participation – do not develop spontaneously (as a kind of social maturation process). They can only be achieved by broadening the 'field of development'. To be able to achieve these, expressly normative, goals, children are continually dependent on the care of adults; they find themselves in a transitional zone 'in which their independence grows gradually, and in which adults help them to gain experience and develop skills' (Elbers, 1993, page 99). According to Elbers, this transitional phase is characterized by 'dependent independence': although the child assumes ever more independent behaviour and judgement, it is at the same time, in view of the complexity of social rules and structures, always dependent on some kind of support from adults. When children are given insufficient stimuli, opportunity or support to open up new horizons in a direction that is meaningful and understandable for them, there is a danger that at an early age they will lose their motivation to learn and act in a responsible way. Greater social participation by children in their direct living environment could constitute a link between abstract learning and the need to explore the outside world; or the need, that basically all children have, to develop into competent, valued and influential members of the community.

Participation and family upbringing

What about the possibilities for children's participation within (and outside) the context of the contemporary family[9]? Does family upbringing provide sufficient opportunities for developing the qualities that are

---

[9]Here we refer to all (primary) lifestyles in which children are cared for and raised.

necessary for participation? The variety in the types of relationships in which children are raised is too great to be able to answer such questions in general terms. Moreover, the way in which children are raised within this wide range of lifestyles is also very diverse. The style of upbringing and the family climate depend, for example, on the socio-economic circumstances, the social status and the educational level of the parents (cf. among others, Jansma, 1988; Janssens & Gerris, 1988). Values and standards that parents use to raise their children are moreover closely related to their cultural background. And yet, scientists regularly try to form absolute, universally valid judgements of child-raising practices in families, on the grounds of empirical research. Such research is then supposed to provide an answer to the question 'what type of upbringing gives the best developmental results in children?'. However, for our subject, answers to this question have very limited usefulness because usually it is only the 'lack of problems and disorders' that is used as a criterion. Part of the developmental psychological research described in the previous section can be classified in this category. In the previously mentioned study by Dekovic et al., for example, the conclusion drawn 'on the basis of clinical impressions' is that parents who ill-treat and/or neglect their children reason at a lower (social–cognitive) level. For this reason, the researchers want to look into the possibilities of helping parents reason in a 'more mature, more child-oriented, more process-oriented way about the parent–child relationship' (Dekovic et al., 1989, page 213). In a recent review article by Scholte and Sontag (1992) we come across a similar approach to the problem. These authors compare a large number of studies on the relation between parental and childhood behaviour. On the grounds of this research they conclude that a democratic or authoritative style of upbringing[10] gives the best results in terms of development. Children who are brought up in such a climate have greater social and cognitive competence, are more independent, and have more self-control than their peers who were brought up along the lines of a pedagogically 'lower' style. And here too, these qualities are rated on the basis of their (assumed) problem-inhibiting potential. The assumption that this western, middle-class ideal also represents an absolute standard for 'good upbringing and development', leads the authors to propose that parents be screened for incompetent and ineffective upbringing behaviour, and that they should be induced to 'better' patterns by the provision of guidance[11].

---

[10]In family research, four different styles of upbringing are often distinguished, namely an authoritarian, a permissive, an absent, and an authoritative or democratic style (cf. Maccoby & Martin, 1983).

[11]The results of this study were strongly criticized by Hermanns (1994) because the authors attribute an absolute value to the data that was collected primarily from middle-class families. He justly accuses them of a lack of 'educational, sociological, cultural or human relativism', by which they imply that educators with other value and norm patterns are incompetent.

In itself it is legitimate for researchers to work on the basis of ideals with respect to upbringing and development. However, in doing so, they take it upon themselves to make these values explicit and to put them into perspective. An apparently neutral appeal to health, balanced or optimal development is not enough. After all, we are talking here about criteria that reflect the extent of adaptation to an existing developmental environment (cf. the views of Bronfenbrenner mentioned on page 59). The question we raise here is a different one. Does the environment offer children sufficient space to orient themselves to society, to be committed to processes in society that are relevant to them and to prepare them for a future role as committed and judicious citizens? In order to answer this question, we have to look at the current family environment for upbringing and development in a somewhat broader context.

In *The making of the modern family*, Shorter (1975) describes the changes that have occurred in western family life since the beginning of the nineteenth century. Although the nature and rate of these changes varies greatly for different social strata, the general trend is that the family, in the course of the modernization process, has become more introverted. In the context of the industrial revolution, it gradually lost its economic–productive function, and acquired more the character of a caring institution. Both the relation between the family and the outside world, and the internal relationships changed as a result. While the gap between the family and the community widened, and was even declared a standard for a good family life, the family members became more mutually dependent. The most important task of the family was now to offer care, warmth and protection, particularly to children. van Setten (1987) speaks of 'the cultivation of emotions'. On the one hand, the modern family became oriented to channelling and controlling affections that previously had been less restrained. On the other, a strong sense of individuality developed and the nature of family upbringing changed as a result. While parents had for a long time provided for the transfer of both knowledge and emotions (many children learned their trades in the 'family business'), the modernization process brought about a division of tasks. The community (namely the educational system) assumed responsibility for the cultivation of knowledge, the family for the cultivation of the emotions (ibid., page 163). With this division of tasks, the world of children became, as it were, divided between family and state. The space that was available for young people to move freely in society has thus become smaller and smaller. Which is not to say that we should idealize the space that they had before. The period in which large groups of children were detained in factories from early morning to late at night for a meagre wage, cannot be typified as a paradise of social orientation. But, in general, the division between the family and public life has made it more difficult for children to prepare themselves practically for adulthood and integration into the community. From an educational point of view, van den Dungen (1989) considers this development to be a serious decline. This division of tasks has meant that parents have become solely responsible for the upbringing of the children, and that children have no example other than the secluded world of the family. 'Previously, children had space around them to explore the world through people they could fit in with and whose art of living they could copy – in both a mental and a material sense. Now they have only their parents' (ibid., page 172). van den Dungen is of the opinion that this isolation (he calls the modern family a 'hotbed of tension') results in disregard for children. They miss having a 'habitat, a familiar ecological space in which they can move about without physical or emotional barriers, and in which they can learn to communicate in a satisfying way with their fellow men'. The result of this, according to van den Dungen, is that when children leave the family they land directly in the big, unfriendly world. 'What is missing is a liveable buffer zone between the private sphere and the world community' (ibid., page 175)[12].

Thus, between the family and the community, there is a space lacking in which actual social orientation can take place through participation[13]. But at the same time, we see that in certain categories of families, the extent of children's participation is actually increasing steadily. Among other things, this has to do with the changing patterns of conduct between parents and children that are typified by de Swaan (1979) as the transition from a commanding household to a negotiating household. The hierarchical differences between parents and children have become smaller, particularly in middle-class families, and with this young people have acquired greater freedom to voice their needs within the family. These days, parents and children often take important family decisions together and, in doing so, have at least the ideal of respecting each other's wishes and needs. Brinkgreve and de Regt (1990) ascribe this change to the progressing emotionality and individualization of family relationships. Raising children has become more psychological, a process in which it is not the 'interests of the family' that constitute the decisive factor, but honouring the needs and interests of individuals, also those of the children. A recent research project in which children and mothers were interviewed (du Bois-Reymond *et al.*, 1992) has shown that a negotiating culture within the family is widespread: most children decide about the arrangement of their rooms, about the way

---

[12]To fill this gap, van den Dungen makes a case for scaling down by revaluing the neighbourhood and organizing communes; children should be able to experience what is happening around them as concretely as possible, so that they are less dependent on 'abstract explanations and joining in at a distance'. Although the author likes this kind of argument, it sounds rather idealistic to him. Such an ideal probably has little to offer young people waiting for its realization.

[13]The question of why schools barely fulfil this function is discussed in Chapter 5.

they spend their leisure time, about their friendships, themselves. If conflicts occur, these are usually resolved by talking things over, and in this children are taught from an early age to motivate their behaviour and put forward their arguments. However, this 'ideal' also calls for a few critical comments. According to Janssen and de Hart (1993), the negotiating culture in families does not necessarily mean that conflicts between parents and children are actually resolved: 'the members of the family accept and understand one another, and accept every difference of opinion, at least, this is the situation in most families' (page 335). This tends to prevent emotional tension from developing rather than resolving it through negotiation. The authors see this avoidance strategy as one of the few options for maintaining close-knit, mutual ties in a rapidly changing culture in which the individual interests of members of the family are becoming increasingly important.

Summarizing, we can say that the present family context both facilitates and impedes the possibilities for children's participation. The modernization of the family culture has resulted in a democratic style of upbringing that has become the norm, and that is gradually spreading to more layers of the population. Within this modern style of upbringing, values such as independence, respect for the opinion of others, and sensitivity to problems play an important role. Whether children actually do learn to negotiate in this climate, or whether they only learn to avoid conflicts is difficult to say. In any case, children, more frequently than in the past, are involved in decisions that are taken within the family. This in itself can be seen as a form of children's participation, but particularly as an important learning experience that can make participation in other relationships possible. But, on the other hand, this same family is an impediment to the greater social commitment of children. It is precisely through processes such as emotionalization and individualization that the attention of the members of the family is directed inwardly, even more than in the past. Intimate relationships between members of the family, particularly between parents and children, are becoming increasingly important and stronger, while the fulfilment of individual needs seems to have been raised to a kind of family ideology. The gap between this closed community of emotionally tied individuals on the one hand, and an anonymous, barely accessible society on the other, lays bare a socialization problem: in what practical situation can children orient and prepare themselves for their later social functioning?

Conclusions

In this chapter, children's and youth participation has been discussed from the perspective of upbringing and development. We have seen that, at the beginning of this century, social educationalists posited the idea of 'community education' as opposed to (or next to) an individual educational theory inspired by the Enlightenment thinkers. The socialization of upbringing was seen as a social necessity. The educational strength of the family and the community had declined markedly following the breakdown of traditional class society, and was apparently no longer sufficient to bind young people to the existing order. Social–educational measures were to fill the gap. Thus, during the first decades of this century, we see that collective involvement in upbringing developed involving all kinds of institutions, such as child health centres, nursery schools, medical and educational advice centres (in the Netherlands: MOB), and youth clubs. Such interventions can be regarded as attempts at preservation – the threat of revolution is often explicitly stated as an argument. Alternatively they bear witness to a real commitment to children who, as a result of poverty, were leading a marginal existence in every respect. It is from this social–educational way of thinking that, here and there, the idea emerged – inspired by adolescence psychology – that young people needed to be better prepared for their lives in society. We described various initiatives that were taken to achieve self-government and self-regulation by children, among others, those of educational theorists such as Kerschensteiner, Dewey, Makarenko and Korczak, all on the basis of widely diverse ideological goals. After the Second World War, participation as a theme disappeared from educational theory. In the 1970s it enjoyed a brief revival when a plea was put forward for the rights of young people in disadvantaged situations to public consultation, social competence and emancipation. Personalistic pedagogical theory, in which the aim of upbringing was described as 'self-responsible self-determination' (a term coined by Langeveld), however, continued to set the tone. In present-day educational science, the relationship between upbringing and the development of society has dropped into the background. Nor was the interest in this relationship ever very strong in the field of developmental psychology. This is surprising, but it can be explained by the fact that this field has been mainly concerned with research into individual and micro-social determinants of development. Moreover, at a time when the nature–nurture debate had more or less died down, and most developmental psychologists had come to recognize the influence of environmental factors, they continued to regard the social context in which this development takes place primarily as a given fact. An exception to this way of thinking was the work of the so-called cultural–historical school (Vygotsky, 1929). From the 1970s onward, critics such as Kessen, Ingleby and Bronfenbrenner claimed that the development of young people was to be regarded as a social construct, in other words as a product of the social relations, values and standards that had developed in the course of history. In this light, the empirical findings of developmental psychology should be regarded as time and culture-bound phenomena, rather than as universal (that is, generally applicable) truths about children. When research reveals that many young people do not or cannot fulfil moral or cognitive 'developmental tasks', then the obvious conclusion is to find out whether the current social conditions offer sufficient possibilities for realizing such tasks. In Bronfenbrenner's terms, offering greater possibilities for orientation and participation could be taken as an ecological experiment to find out whether broadening the 'developmental field' does actually result in other developmental outcomes. In this way, all kinds of 'shortcomings' that are readily ascribed to young people these days, such as a lack of social responsibility, the decay of moral principles, and materialism, may come to be seen in a totally different light. We stated that the stimulation and support of social participation could fill the gap between the abstract nature of learning processes and the fundamental human need to function in a socially competent and meaningful way.

In the last section, we described one of the main factors that go to make up the developmental profile of young people, namely the relationship between the family and society. While modern family upbringing appears to be developing in a democratic way, we also see an enormous distance between the family and society. As a result of this, there is, as it were, a gap in the socialization process. A social training ground in which skills, competencies and attitudes learned within the family can actually be developed before the child is required to be wholly independent, is lacking. Such training grounds do exist potentially: local youth policy, education and all kinds of youth care could in principle offer sufficient possibilities for this. But if these contexts are to actually fulfil a function of education in citizenship, then young people have to be given the chance to participate in them. Therefore, in the chapters that follow, we look at these sectors from that perspective.

References

Abma R (1993) Jeugdonderzoek in Nederland. In: AJ Dieleman, FJ van der Linden & AC Perreijn (red) *Jeugd in meervoud*. Utrecht/Heerlen: Tijdstroom & Open Universiteit, pp. 85–101.

Bavinck H (1916) *De opvoeding der rijpere jeugd*. Kampen: JH Kok.

Bertels K (1978a) Adolescentie als historisch maakwerk. *Jeugd en Samenleving*, 8. pp. 17–34.

Bertels K (1978b) Puberteit als historisch maakwerk. *Jeugd en Samenleving*, 8. pp. 263–82.

Bois-Reymond M du, D de Ruiter & I Steffens (1992) *Onderhandelingsculturen in gezinnen. Een onderzoek naar verzelfstandigingsprocessen van kinderen*. RU Leiden: Sectie Jongerenstudies en Jeugdbeleid.

Bremner JG (1987) *Infancy*. Oxford: Blackwell.

Brinkgreve C & A de Regt (1990) Het verdwijnen van de vanzelfsprekendheid. Over de gevolgen van individualisering voor kinderen. *Jeugd en Samenleving*, jrg. 20, nr. 5/6. pp. 324–33.

Bronfenbrenner U (1979a) *The ecology of human development*. Cambridge, Mass: Harvard University Press.

Bronfenbrenner U (1979b) De experimentele ecologie van de menselijke ontwikkeling. In: W Koops & JJ van der Werff (red) *Overzicht van de ontwikkelingspsychologie*. Groningen: Wolters-Noordhof. pp. 407–23.

Bruner J (1977) Early social interaction and language acquisition. In: HR Schaffer (ed) *Studies in mother–infant interaction*. Cambridge: Cambridge University Press. pp. 271–89.

Carpay JAM (1994) *Een school voor toekomstige burgers*. Tekst van de derde Langeveld-lezing gehouden op 20-4-1994. Utrecht: ISOR.

Coumou H & W van Stegeren (1987) Sociale pedagogiek in historisch perspectief. In: J Hazekamp & I van der Zande (red) *Jongeren. Nieuwe wegen in de sociale pedagogiek*. Meppel: Boom. pp. 35–49.

Damon W (1988) *The moral child. Nurturing children's natural moral growth*. New York: The Free Press.

Dasberg L (1975) *Groot brengen door klein houden als historisch verschijnsel*. Meppel: Boom (gebruikt elfde druk 1986).

Dasberg L (1993) *Meelopers en dwarsliggers*. Amsterdam/Hoevelaken: Trouw & Christelijk Pedagogisch Studiecentrum.

Dekovic M, JMA Janssens & JRM Gerris (1989) Niveaus van redeneren over ouder-kind relatie, ouderlijke gedragingen en de sociaal–cognitieve ontwikkeling van het kind. *Gezin*, jrg. 1, nr. 4. pp. 201–14.

Dennis W (1972) Historical beginnings of child psychology. In: W Dennis (ed) *Historical readings in developmental psychology*. New York: Appleton-Century-Crofts. pp. 222–35.

Dibbits Tj (1987) Jongeren in cultuurhistorisch perspectief. In: J Hazekamp & I van der Zande (red) *Jongeren. Nieuwe wegen in de sociale pedagogiek*. Meppel: Boom. pp. 17–35.

Diekstra RFW (1992) De adolescentie: biologische, psychologische en sociale aspecten. In: RFW Diekstra (ed) *Jeugd in ontwikkeling*. 's-Gravenhage: SDU. pp. 111–57.

Donaldson M (1978) *Children's minds*. London: Fontana Paperbacks.

Dungen M van den (1989) Het broeikaseffect: gezin en samenleving rond 2000. *Gezin*, jrg. 1, nr. 3. pp. 164–80.

Elbers EPJ (1988) *Social context and the child's construction of knowledge*.

Dissertatie Rijksuniversiteit Utrecht.

Elbers EPJ (1993) De verschuivende zone tussen zorg en zelfstandigheid. Een ontwikkelingspsychologisch perspectief. In: C van Nijnatten (ed) *Kinderrechten in discussie*. Meppel: Boom. pp. 81–101.

Emde RN & JF Sorce (1983) The rewards of infancy: Emotional availability and maternal referencing. In: JD Call ea (eds) *Frontiers of infant psychiatry*. New York: Basic Books. pp. 17–30.

Gesell A (1928) *Infancy and human growth*. New York: Macmillan.

Goodman WL (1949) *Anton Simeonovitch Makarenko. Russian Teacher*. London: Routledge & Kegan Paul Ltd.

Graaf WAW de (1989) *De zaaitijd bij uitnemendheid. Jeugd en puberteit in Nederland 1900–1940*. Dissertatie Rijksuniversiteit Leiden. Academisch Boekencentrum.

Hall GS (1904) *Adolescence. Its psychology and its relations to physiology, anthropology, sociology, sex, crime, religion and education*. New York: Appleton.

Harmsen G (1961) *Blauwe en rode jeugd. Ontstaan, ontwikkeling en teruggang van de Nederlandse jeugdbeweging tussen 1853 en 1940*. Assen: Van Gorcum & Comp.

Hart RA (1992) *Children's participation. From tokenism to citizenship*. Florence, UNICEF Innocenti Essays nr. 4.

Hazekamp JL, J van der Gauw & J Nuijens (1993) *Jongeren doen mee aan beleid. Verslag van een onderzoek naar politieke participatie van jongeren op lokaal niveau*. 's-Gravenhage: VNG.

Hermanns JMA (1994) Bespreking van EM Scholte & L Sontag: Opvoeding en ontwikkeling. *Jeugd en Samenleving*, nr. 2, februari. pp. 115–17.

Hessen JS van (1965) *Samen jong zijn*. Assen: Van Gorcum/Prakke.

Heymans PG (1992) Moraliteit: competenties en ontwikkelingstaken. In: RFW Diekstra (ed) *Jeugd in ontwikkeling*. 's-Gravenhage: SDU. pp. 157–201.

Ijzendoorn MH van (1985) De gehechtheidstheorie, over de levensloop van een onderzoeksprogramma voor vroegkinderlijke opvoeding en ontwikkeling. In: J de Wit, HJ Groenedaal & JM van Meel (eds) *Psychologen over het kind, 8*. Lisse: Swets & Zeitlinger. pp. 55–78.

Ingleby JD (1986) Development in social context. In: P Light & M Richards (eds) *Children in social worlds*. Cambridge: Polity Press.

Ingleby JD & PP Goudena (1992) Raakvlakken en spanningen tussen psychoanalyse en ontwikkelingspsychologie. In: CHJ van Nijnatten (red) *Psychodynamische ontwikkelingsmodellen*. Meppel: Boom. pp. 166–96.

Jansma JBM (1988) *Gezinsklimaat, een onderzoek naar het gezinsklimaat bij gezinnen met en gezinnen zonder opvoedingsproblemen m.b.v. de gezinsklimaatschaal.* Dissertatie Rijksuniversiteit Utrecht.

Janssen JAP & JJM de Hart (1993) Religie en levensbeschouwing. In: AJ Dieleman, FJ van der Linden & AC Perreijn (red) *Jeugd in meervoud.* Utrecht/Heerlen: Tijdstroom & Open Universiteit. pp. 326–39.

Janssens, JMA & JRM Gerris (1988) Sociaal milieu en reacties van ouders op disciplineringssituaties: een empirisch verklaringsmodel. *Pedagogische Studieën,* jrg. **65,** nr. 5. pp. 185–97.

Kaye K (1982) *The mental and social life of babies. How parents create persons.* Chicago: The University of Chicago Press.

Kerschensteiner G (1917) *Staatsbürgerliche Erziehung der deutschen Jugend.* Erfurt (zesde druk).

Kessen W (1983) The child and other cultural inventions. In: F Kessel & AW Siegel (eds) *The child and other cultural inventions.* New York: Praeger. pp. 27–39.

Kohlberg L (1979) De continuïteit in de morele ontwikkeling: een herbezinning. In: W Koops & JJ van der Werff (red) *Overzicht van de ontwikkelingspsychologie.* Groningen: Wolters-Noordhof. pp. 307–25.

Kohlberg L (1985) The just community in theory and practice. In: M Berkowitz & F Oser (eds) *Moral education.* Hillsdale, NJ: Erlbaum.

Kohnstamm Ph (1919) *Staatspaedagogiek of persoonlijkheidspaedagogiek.* Groningen/DenHaag: Wolters.

Korczak J (1920) *Jak Kochac Dzieco.* Nederlandse vertaling: *Hoe houd je van een kind.* Utrecht, Bijleveld, 1986.

Kuipers HJ (1992) *De wereld als werkplaats. Over de vorming van Kees Boeke en Beatrice Cadbury.* Amsterdam: IISG.

Maccoby EE & JA Martin (1983) Socialization in the context of the family: parent–child interaction. In: PH Mussen (ed) *Handbook of Child-Psychology,* Vol. 4, Socialization, personality, and social development. New York: Wiley. pp. 1–101.

Mahler MS, F Pine & A Bergman (1975) *The psychological birth of the human infant.* New York: Basic Books.

Mahler MS (1983) The meaning of developmental research of earliest infancy as related to the study of separation–individuation. In: JD Call ea (eds) *Frontiers of infant psychiatry.* New York: Basic Books. pp. 3–7.

Mennicke CA (1937) *Sociale pedagogie. Grondslagen, vormen en middelen der gemeenschapsopvoeding.* Utrecht: Erven J. Bijleveld.

Miedema S & MH van Ijzendoorn (1992) Pedagogiek temidden van de sociale wetenschappen. In: AJ Dielema & P Span (red) *Pedagogiek van de levensloop*. Amersfoort/Leuven: ACCO. pp. 258–68.

Mollenhauer K (1986) *Vergeten samenhang. Over cultuur en opvoeding*. Meppel: Boom.

Natorp P (1899) *Sozialpädagogik. Theorie der willenserziehung auf der grundlage der gemeinschaft*. Stuttgart (vierde druk 1920).

Noordman J & H van Setten (1989) De ontwikkeling van de ouder/kind-verhouding in het gezin. In: HFM Peeters, L Dresen-Coenders & T Brandenburg (red) *Vijf eeuwen gezinsleven. Liefde, huwelijk en opvoeding in Nederland*. Nijmegen: SUN. pp. 140–62.

Parreren CF van (1979) Onderzoek van de cognitieve ontwikkeling in de Sovjetunie. In: W Koops & JJ van der Werff (red) *Overzicht van de ontwikkelingspsychologie*. Groningen: Wolters-Noordhof. pp. 195–214.

Peeters J & C Woldringh (1993) *Leefsituatie van kinderen tot 12 jaar in Nederland*. Nijmegen: ITS.

Piaget J (1923, 1955) *The language and thought of the child*. London: Routledge & Kegan Paul. (Uitg. 1955 Meridian Books, New York).

Piaget J (1963) *The origins of intelligence in children*. New York: Norton.

Röling HQ (1982) Onderwijs in Nederland. In: B Kruithof, J Noordman & P de Rooy (red) *Geschiedenis van opvoeding en onderwijs. Inleiding bronne-nonderzoek*. pp. 66–86. Nijmegen: SUN.

Rooy P de (1982) Jeugdbeweging in Nederland. In: B Kruithof, J Noordman & P de Rooy (red) *Geschiedenis van opvoeding en onderwijs. Inleiding bronnenonderzoek*. pp. 127–38. Nijmegen: SUN.

Sameroff AJ (1975) Early influences on development: Fact or fancy. *Merill Palmer Quarterly*, Vol. 21, nr. 4. pp. 267–94.

Scholte EM & L Sontag (1992) *Opvoeding en ontwikkeling. Een litera-tuuronderzoek naar de samenhang tussen opvoedingsgedrag van primaire opvoeders en de ontwikkeling van jeugdigen*. Utrecht: PCOJ.

Selman RL (1976) Toward a structural analysis of developing interpersonal relations concepts: Research with normal and disturbed preadolescent boys. In: A Pack (ed) *Tenth Annual Minnesota Symposium on Child Psychology*. Minneapolis: University of Minnesota Press. pp. 156–200.

Selten PJH (1991) *Het apostolaat der jeugd. Katholieke jeugdbewegingen in Nederland 1900–1941*. Dissertatie K.U.N.

Setten H van (1987) *In de schoot van het gezin: opvoeding in Nederlandse gezinnen in de twintigste eeuw*. Nijmegen: SUN.

Shorter E (1975) *The making of the modern family*. New York: Basic Books.

Singer E (1989) *Kinderopvang en de moeder-kindrelatie. Pedagogen, psychologen en sociale hervormers over moeders en jonge kinderen.* Van Loghum Slaterus. Dissertatie RU Utrecht.

Skolnick A (1976) Introduction: Rethinking childhood. In: A. Skolnick (ed) *Rethinking childhood. Perspectives on development and society.* Boston/ Toronto: Little, Brown & Company.

Sommerville CJ (1982) *The rise and fall of childhood.* Beverly Hills: Sage Publications.

Stern DN, RK Barnett & S Spieker (1983) Early transmission of affect: Some research issues. In: JD Call ea (eds) *Frontiers of infant psychiatry.* New York: Basic Books. pp. 74–83.

Stone LJ, H Smith & LB Murphy (1973) *The competent infant.* New York: Basic Books.

Swaan A de (1979) *Uitgaansbeperkingen en uitgangsangst. Over de verschuiving van bevelshuishouding naar onderhandelingshuishouding.* Amsterdam: Meulenhoff.

Thorndike EL (1913) *The original nature of man.* New York: Teachers College.

Valsiner J (1987) *Culture and the development of children's action.* Chichester: Wiley.

Vermeer ALR (1987) *Philipp A Kohnstamm over democratie.* Proefschrift Rijksuniversiteit Utrecht. Kampen: Kok.

Vygotsky LS (1929) The problem of the cultural development of the child. *Journal of Genetic Psychology*, **36.** pp. 415–34.

Watson JB (1925) *Behaviorism.* New York: Norton.

Winter M de (1986) *Het voorspelbare kind. VTO (vroegtijdige onderkenning van ontwikkelingsstoornissen) in wetenschappelijk en sociaal-historisch perspectief.* Lisse: Swets & Zeitlinger. Dissertatie Katholieke Universiteit Brabant.

Part Two

Participation and local youth policy

Introduction

Children and young people are not only educated in the secluded world of home and school. In Bronfenbrenner's terms, their development is largely determined by their functioning in meso-, exo-, and macro-systems (cf. page 59). This idea has far-reaching implications. It actually means that the education of young people takes place everywhere and all the time, so also in social contexts which we in our day generally do not consider to be exactly educational. When a municipal official or a community worker organizes a dialogue with children to talk to them about safety in the neighbourhood or its liveability – and certainly if such a dialogue has visible consequences – then this is an educational activity. Because in this way, children do not only learn 'technical' skills such as negotiating, balancing of interests and cooperation, but are particularly imparted something about the relationship between themselves and 'society'. As a child or young person you are appreciated, your opinion is considered to be of importance and on the other hand it appears that hidden behind local authorities or official bodies there are people with democratic ideas who need actively involved recipients if they are to pursue good policy. But the reverse applies too; when all kinds of provisions for young people are made in a neighbourhood without them having been involved themselves, then you are implicitly given to understand – even if it isn't meant that way – that you as a child don't actually amount to much. The educational message is that an anonymous body (the local authority) apparently has the best intentions regarding children (after all, a safe cycle path has been provided), but that the children's point of view has not played a role of any importance. Thus a contribution is made to the creation of a citizen with little competence, who has learnt since childhood that society consists of those who have responsibility, and those who do not.

In brief, whether society wants to or not, whether it acts consciously or not, it educates the young. This idea may not be easily absorbed into the vocabulary of the educationalists, who only call education education when it takes place with 'deliberation' (cf. Imelman, 1974; Faber, 1987). Such a restriction has more to do with the scientific and professional identity of the discipline than with the everyday reality in which children grow up. For the educational role which local youth policy plays in the lives of children and young people is not to be underestimated. In Dutch municipalities a great number of activities are undertaken that are aimed at directly influencing this group of the public. We are thinking here of policy sectors such as welfare, public health, education, social services and public order. Social education takes place, either implicitly or explicitly in each of these fields. The way in which children and young people are approached by those in authority, policy-makers, official bodies, professionals or volunteers, contributes to the image they form of society and their own role within it. This is why it is very important that a lot of thought is given to the educational implications of local youth policy. We shall not be able to go into all the aspects of local youth policy in this chapter. Nor can we consider in detail the specific methods that are applied in local policy. Here we are particularly concerned with the question of how local policy contributes to the 'education for citizenship'. Again, the starting point is that social interventions directed at the young have by definition a formative character. Putting high railings with spikes around a community centre that is susceptible to vandalism makes it clear to the young that they are indeed being taken seriously, as a hostile group. This simply challenges them to demolish the railings. Conversely, arranging a discussion and offering possibilities for joint responsibility is more than just vandalism prevention: it is an approach that values the young for their abilities and stimulates them towards social commitment.

A child-forgotten place to live

'Children also live somewhere', the educationalists Bleeker and Mulderij wrote in the early 1980s. The studies they did (1982) on the way children experience their 'child-forgotten neighbourhoods' drew attention to the fact that the way post-war society had tried to solve its housing shortages and lack of space had not favoured children. Their expressive descriptions of children's lives in large scale high-rise estates, new growth centres, old working-class districts and country villages present a picture of a society which whilst striving towards economic growth has forgotten the interests and needs of its children. High-rise flats restrain young children's urge to explore; respectable newly built estates are boring because of the rift between dwelling and working, the sterility of the laid out playgrounds and the fact that there is nothing going on for the older children; in old urban areas parked cars and cycles have taken over much of the children's space; and in the country the sense of safety is treacherous, because the traffic is getting steadily heavier and faster. 'Children are not well served by the neat-and-tidiness and the separation of functions in our residential areas. This leads to deterioration of the opportunities for play and adventure and possibly, in the worst case, to aggression' say the authors (ibid., page 25). The many suggestions they made to improve the situation amounted to tailoring residential surroundings to child size. To be able to understand the perception children have of the world, and then to draw the correct conclusions in furnishing these surroundings, 'pedagogy must be carried out on its knees'; the educationalist seen as an advocate and interpreter of children's interests (cf. Bleeker & Mulderij, 1984).

Such a plea did not come out of a clear blue sky. The quality and quantity of children's space in residential areas had never had a very high priority in the policies of the various authorities. They were happy to leave this aspect to private initiative, such as the many associations that had been established in the Netherlands from the beginning of the century to create play and recreation facilities for the young, in the context of advancing urbanization. It is only quite recently that the disinterested attitude of authorities seems to have changed. This is not so much the result of spontaneously blossoming child-friendliness, but rather of a markedly changing situation on the housing market. Now that the worst housing shortages in the Netherlands are over, thanks to large scale building in the 1970s and 1980s, local authorities and housing associations are operating in a competitive market. The 'housing wishes of the housing consumer' now suddenly play an important role. The battle for his favours has placed items such as residential surroundings, traffic safety and recreational facilities high on the agenda. There is a wish to draw up the improvement plans for neighbourhoods and districts, which include defining the interaction between children, playing and public housing, in consultation with younger as well as adult residents. A recent statement by a representative of the housing associations during a congress on playground policy is characteristic: 'Associations developing neighbourhood improvement plans will have to take serious account, even if only on the basis of economic motives, of those for whom the neighbourhood is intended. And if the chosen target group is families, then planners' ideas will have to be centred on children, so that a liveable world is achieved for them too. If an association does not do this, it will be damaging to both the development of children and its own pocket, because today's housing consumer tenaciously demands this' (Sturkenboom, 1993).

Children's participation and the layout of public space

The idea of also involving children when planning a neighbourhood is not entirely new. As early as the beginning of the 1980s, when notions such as public consultation and having a voice had become good form, a plea for 'consultation of children' was heard from various sides, especially in regard to play facilities in a neighbourhood. The NUSO, a national organization for playground work and youth recreation, issued a brochure in 1984 in which participation was described not as a favour for children but as their right: 'Mr Government should really say thank-you to you kids for wanting to think and talk about what the place you are going to live in should look like; then at least we won't be making a neighbourhood where everyone will be having nervous breakdowns because of the noise, or where children will be killed on the roads every other day' (NUSO, 1984). It is apparent from this text that there was a lot of opposition from policy-makers and residents of the neighbourhoods. An appendix comprised an extensive list of 'prejudices' against child consultation. Clearly there were the objections that children would not be able to cope with the responsibility, that they would not be able to judge the consequences of decisions, and that child consultation was an illusion because legally they had no say. At that time there were few positive examples to counter these. The brochure only contains one case of consultation concerning opportunities for play. In the years following the issue of the brochure, children's participation hardly took any hold on local youth policy.

A first personal introduction to children's participation, or rather the almost entire lack of it, dates from 1992. The author was then a jury member for the competition 'Youth City Predicate', to choose the most child- and youth-friendly local authority in the Netherlands. What has endured in his memory from the early jury meetings is the deluging amount of paper on which about 50 participating authorities presented their provisions and plans for the target group as favourably as possible. 'Integrated youth policy, coherence in provisions, prevention, care-to-measure, teenage hangouts, traffic constraining measures, creative play opportunities, graffiti-tolerated zones'. It must be said, many Dutch municipalities put their best foot forward as far as the young are concerned. Yet there was a strange vacuum concealed in almost all the entries. There was hardly a whisper of the opinions of children and young people. It seemed as though in Holland most local policy for the young came into being without the young. However, there were a few positive exceptions. Some local authorities had really involved children in the design and implementation of provisions such as play areas and traffic measures. They had done painstaking work, with more or less success it must be said, on dialogues with children and young people. And it had paid off. Children were enthusiastic because somebody listened to them. The playground that they had helped to design and draw had really turned out to be their own playground. Parents and other adult neighbourhood residents were enthusiastic as, because of their greater commitment the young were far less destructive. And the local authorities had discovered just what they wanted. Actively involving the young had proved not only to be an effective way of implementing youth policy, but also a possible lead to forms of efficient neighbourhood policy and prevention of vandalism. Meanwhile this trend seems to be making headway on a larger scale. More and more local authorities see active involvement of children (and parents) in planning public spaces as a means of improving the liveability of the so-called problem neighbourhoods. The Netherlands Council for Youth Policy published a report in 1993 in which a great number of examples of this trend are discussed (Visser, 1993). Child consultation is being used much more often as 'a tool to get children's ideas, wishes and hankerings into the open and to use the structural information about their play space which only children can give in the different phases of a neighbourhood renewal' (NUSO, 1993). Children are asked to discuss wishes and possibilities amongst themselves and with designers. They make sketch plans, they construct models and finally, where possible, they are involved in the implementation of the plans. This is an example from Amsterdam:

> *Souad Kasmi is 11 years old. She goes to the Vogelnest School in North Amsterdam. Together with about 20 children from her school and other nearby schools she sat on the children's neighbourhood council that, guided by Jaap Bros (the designer, Micha de Winter), made a complete design for the Play Park on a city square. The only objective that was laid down beforehand was that something was needed for the six- to twelve-year-olds. 'We met often, six or seven times I think; it took five weeks altogether. Usually we talked and made plans and drawings. Mr Jaap Bros was always there. When we had made a park he told us why some things couldn't be done. Like when some of us wanted paving and some wanted grass. Well, you couldn't have both. And then we talked about that. And we wanted a castle and that might be too expensive. Then we had to think of something else that was cheaper. We made three or four parks. I thought it was great fun. And at the end we got a diploma because we had taken part. It's hanging on the wall at home.' The entire project was realized in nine months, from the first discussion with the children to completion. Even the castle was there, although it was a cheaper version than the one the children had thought up (NUSO, ibid.).*

The examples mentioned here come from fairly clear-cut, small scale projects. The city of Utrecht has for some time wanted to incorporate children's participation in municipal policy. In 1992 the city council passed a resolution stating that from then on every council proposal must include a youth section. This should indicate the consequences for children and young people of plans in the fields of public open space, traffic, housing, or economic activities. Such plans should also indicate in what way the young will be involved. Throughout the city, children's conferences were held in which administrators and councillors talked to children about the wishes they had for their neighbourhoods, wishes which they had already been able to bring forward in a questionnaire[1]. Has Utrecht suddenly discovered the child as a fellow citizen? This is far from certain. The city council took this step particularly because it had serious worries, heightened by social and economic motives, about the exodus from the city, particularly by families with young children. But whatever the true motives may have been, Utrecht is the first large city in the Netherlands that made child participation a policy spearhead. It was notably for this reason that Utrecht was awarded the Youth City Predicate in 1994.

The initiatives of local authorities to actively involve children in provisions for the residential environment, mentioned above, seem therefore to have gained their chance mainly due to the discovery that children are an item in the local cashbook. In spite of the undoubtedly favourable effect that the rising appreciation of children's participation in this field can have on the quality of the lives of both children and parents, a little scepticism is called for. The involvement of children in municipal policy still has a specifically 'instrumental' reason, namely the achievement in the short term of policy aims that are sensitive to economic fluctuations. These include neighbourhood policy and neighbourhood crime prevention, enhancement of the residential environment, the avoidance of mass departures and of unoccupied houses. For the children involved the motivation behind it all is of little importance; they have gained worthwhile experience, have felt respected and even seen some upshot of their efforts. However important the arguments mentioned may be, if participation is to become a stable element of policy, recognition of the surplus educational value is needed. In the various evaluations and descriptions of processes, hardly any attention has been paid to the educational side of the matter. Careful charting of the educational effects is however extremely necessary, not only to enable improvement of the methodological quality of such projects, but especially to let society see that children's participation can represent a true contribution to education and socialization. When houses are once again easy to let, and when the city no longer feels threatened by mass departures and impoverishment, it will be just as important to educate children to social commitment.

A specific form of participation which warrants a mention here is that of

---

[1]At a conference which the author attended the children did a lot better than the administrators; they posed crystal-clear questions and made concrete proposals. The Mayor's answers were very much vaguer; his repertory mainly consisted of 'we'll give that some consideration' and 'shall we agree that you try to do something about it yourself'. The boy who would like some more trees on his road didn't seem to find this much help, nor did the girl who asked 'you must be high-up, can you see to it that the postman doesn't always piss in our gallery?' Child participation sometimes appears harder for adults than for children!

the children's and youth councils functioning in a number of municipalities. Some have been set up round specific activities or projects, others have a more permanent character and cover the whole field of local youth policy (Salman, 1993). An example of the first type is that in Schiedam. In the framework of the campaign 'Schiedammers from everywhere and nowhere', launched in 1991 to generate more mutual understanding between the various population groups in the city, all primary schools were asked if they would appoint representatives to a children's local council. This move was inspired by the traditional Turkish 'Day of the Child'. The assignment for the children's council was to design a new play area in the municipality. Locations were inspected, sketches and models made, and finally the children chose the best plan. However there were a lot of difficulties with the actual implementation. After the children's council had made its choice it appeared that three of the locations the municipality had designated were unsuitable, so new ones had to be sought and new designs made. Nevertheless, the authorities were so enthusiastic that it has been decided to install a children's council every year, with a different assignment each time (Visser, 1993). A number of Dutch municipalities have a youth council with a wide-ranging advisory function. Young people of between 15 and 30 years of age constitute a board that gives solicited or unsolicited recommendations to the municipality about its policy for children and the young. Salman (1993) is more positive about the youth councils on a project basis than about such advisory boards. In particular, the tangible results in councils of the first type prove very stimulating for young people. Especially due to the involvement of schools, they can make much larger groups of children enthusiastic. The impression gained of the permanent boards is that they quickly become entangled in local politics. The decision-making process is often unclear to young people because their recommendations are passed on to the municipal executive and they lose sight of the further process.

In France the idea of young people's local councils has been widely accepted since 1979 (the International Year of the Child). Currently about 650 municipalities have such councils. The members are usually between 9 and 18 years of age and are elected from schools. They have their own budget and they develop projects related to themes like culture and leisure, solidarity (between the various ethnic groups) and safety in the community. A national organization has been set up which provides support, furnishes information to municipalities and council members and arranges gatherings (ANACEJ, 1992). International exchanges also take place with increasing regularity with Italy, Portugal, Germany, Israel and so on. Although the organization emphasizes education for citizenship (éducation civique), a preventive effect is also attributed to the councils. The French National Council for the Prevention of Criminality sees this as a new approach to counteracting the marginalization of the young.

Participation and integrated youth policy

For a long time youth policy was mainly youth-work policy. The club and community-centre work, nowadays called socio-cultural youth work, originated in society's fear and concern about the development of the young masses, whom the bourgeois circles felt should be converted to 'civilization'. At the turn of the century private individuals set up *Volkshuizen* to keep the working class youth off the streets by providing recreation and education. Because this free youth movement (cf. page 54) failed to catch on, clubhouses with a clearly formative character were set up in numerous towns and villages after the First World War. The working class youth should not only be kept off the streets, they should be educated. After 1945 the concern about the asocial character of the young masses was still evident. From the 1950s the Dutch government took an active interest; it had research done (Langeveld, 1952b), and began to subsidize club and community-centre work to a limited degree. The aim became to educate to mental adulthood, and professional youth workers were to set a good example. In the 1960s and 1970s attempts were made to give club and community-centre work a more independent position. The young had to be supported in obtaining a say in the sectors of society that were relevant to them, such as school and the work floor. As already noted, this politicizing approach had little success with working-class youth. Gradually attention shifted to care and guidance of problem target groups, such as marginalized youth and the young of ethnic minorities. After the introduction of the Social Welfare Act (1989), socio-cultural youth work became the responsibility of the municipalities. Local authorities could now use this type of work as an instrument for their own youth policy. However, they had to cope simultaneously with severe cutbacks in expenditure which had a serious affect on socio-cultural youth work. Yet this youth work still has an important intermediary role in today's local youth policy. Youth workers – for children, teenagers or young adults – often provide the points of contact between the young in the neighbourhoods and the local authority. Youth work has the task of fulfilling the needs of children and young people in regard to worthwhile leisure activities. But it is also involved in improving the future position of young people in society by means of activities aimed at education, emancipation and participation. So in this way, such work is also a kind of municipal educational service.

Recent years have seen a tendency towards broadening local youth policy. More services and authorities have to concern themselves with the young, the doctrine being an integrated approach. The report *The future of municipal youth policy* gives four reasons for this (Bertels *et al.*, 1989, pages 7–8):

1   the increasingly manifest problems among the young, such as truancy, marginalization, juvenile unemployment, vandalism, alcohol and drug addictions, the problems of minorities, and the position of girls with little schooling on the employment market. The current range of provisions does not seem adequately geared to these; the compartmentalization of existing specialisms being a major cause

2   local governments are confronted with these problems in two ways, that is because of the young and youth provisions calling for more funds, and by the public demanding measures against nuisance caused by the young

3   the tasks for local authorities in the field of youth policy are becoming more and more extensive; national government policy is aimed at the prevention of marginalization, which implies on the one hand that problems among the young must be spotted as early as possible, and on the other hand that social care should take place as near as possible to the young people's own social environment. Local provisions such as the socio-cultural work, police, education and social work play an important part

4   the necessity, resulting from cutbacks, to work more efficiently and with greater effect.

Between 1987 and 1991 some twelve Dutch municipalities experimented with integrated youth policy. The aim of these experiments, subsidized by the Ministry of Welfare, Public Health and Cultural Affairs, was 'to achieve a policy at local level that will be able to produce a coherent pattern of provisions, geared to the wishes and needs of the young. Young people themselves should emphatically play a role in the development of this policy'. Although intensifying participation, for instance in regard to the development of their provisions by the young themselves, appears to be the obvious way to implement policy effectively, in practice there prove to be many obstacles to achieving this ideal. In *The young partake in policy*, Hazekamp, van der Gaauw and Nuijens (1993) report on a study concerning the way in which the municipalities involved dealt with the participation issue. The problem thesis was 'in how far and in what way did participation by young people (from the age of approximately 16) in the municipal experiments in integrated youth policy take shape, and under what conditions is it possible for the young to participate in the municipal policy process?'. The investigators distinguish four types of participation, which require a rising degree of activity from the young:

1   *information*: the local authority finds out what its young people's needs are and informs them about its policy

2   *informal consultation*: the local authority organizes consultation meetings so as to listen direct to its young

3 *formal consultation*: the local authority initiates permanent consulta-
tive bodies with the young

4 *participation in decision-making*: young people take part on a basis of
equality in consultations with the local authority.

A striking point in the results is that the investigators could only qualify
one of the more than 50 projects they described as meriting the term
'participation in decision-making'. In all the other projects, young people
were either used as a source of information (for instance via interviews or
questionnaires), were informed about the policy intentions of the local
authority (via the local media or the schools), or were 'given a hearing' via
discussions or consultation. The authors sum up numerous factors that
prove to facilitate or to impede the participation of the young. The
enthusiasm of civil servants, administrators and youth workers in making
contact with young people, and their willingness to brave together the often
lengthy trail through municipal bureaucracy and regulations, proved to be
important conditions for the success of the projects. The obstacles were
mainly lack of experience and expertize (on the part of adults as well as of
the young), loss of patience and sometimes dropping out by the young due
to long and complex procedures, and especially the tremendous culture gap
between the young person's perception of the world around him/her and
the world of municipal bureaucracy. A further hindrance was constituted,
in the opinion of the authors, by the prejudices about the young harboured
by decision-makers: i.e. that they would act too much on the basis of self-
interest; would be unable to defer the instant satisfaction of their
requirements. Neither was their competence very highly regarded. As
remarked in the report, 'Not once was there an acknowledgement of those
qualities of young people that could greatly influence municipal youth
policy ... such as originality, creativity, honesty, unexpected points of view
and craftsmanship' (ibid., page 86).

Participation in local policy by young people does not come easy, is the
conclusion. Much resistance and many prejudices have to be overcome,
procedures must be revised, new methods must be developed, the job
descriptions of civil servants and youth workers have to be adapted, they
have to take refresher courses, special attention must be paid to girls and to
the young from ethnic backgrounds, and last but not least – everyone must
want it to succeed. This last situation is already very often the case, the
authors say, amongst both the young and the other actors. So the report
also presents a great many positive experiences with youth participation. If
overcoming the obstacles in a dialogue with the young in a municipality
actually succeeds and, for instance, a provision they want like a skateboard
track, their own news-sheet, a young people's platform, is realized, then
everybody is satisfied; the young because people seriously listened to them,
administrators and civil servants because a negative spiral of nuisance and
its containment could be halted.

An illustration: the case of FC Utrecht

The Dutch city of Utrecht, like many other European cities, has a hard core of young football hooligans, known as the B-side. For a long time, this group had presented a big problem for both FC Utrecht and the city. In general the boys involved receive little social respect and in turn they couldn't care less what society thinks of them. They derive their identity mainly from the colour of their flags and caps, which distinguish them from the enemy who, of course, sport a different combination of colours. And then they have another source of identity and sense of belonging to the group: the immense attention they receive from the media and the police. The number of Utrecht police working overtime for home matches on Sundays rose steadily, as did that of the barricades of skips set up by the municipality every two weeks to separate the various supporter groups. However, something has changed. Nowadays not much is heard of the B-side. The football club came to the conclusion that the boys actually had little else beside their negative supportership, and it decided to risk an attempt at channelling their energy into a positive direction. A hefty, not easy to scare youth-worker was engaged and he approached the hard core of the group, consisting of some 25 youngsters. FC Utrecht made a deal with the group about the management of 'their' section. For some time now they have organized the sale of tickets for this section, they check the tickets, they provide their own attendants and they run their own supporters' home in the bowels of the stadium. In other words they have obtained and have taken up the responsibility for curbing the problems which they themselves bring about; and it is said, with much success. A considerable bond has grown up between the group and the club, and this has had its influence on other youthful supporters. The former hooligans have become, as it were, a positive part of the football circus. Not so long ago such an approach would immediately have been typified and rejected as a form of *repressive tolerance*, as a clever but repressive policy measure. Although the management aspect is certainly there, this approach may be characterized as a classic example of *youth participation*. It is a form of social commitment that is not only positive for society, but certainly also for the young people involved, who have gained in at least two ways. In the first place they have become respectable in the eyes of two bodies that are extremely important to them, the club and the police. And in the second place, although this is still speculation, this development may have a big effect on their self-respect. After all, here is a group of the young (we could call them marginalized young) who have had very little positive social experience in their lives until now.

To summarize, we are concerned here with a fairly simple intervention with possibly far-reaching social and educational effects. A group of young people whose problematic aspects have thus far almost always been addressed, and for whom greater repression only created an increasingly greater challenge, have been approached the other way round. Adults have addressed their capacities, their desire to amount to something in society. In short, the problem approach has been replaced by a participation approach.

The young scientist

Local youth policy is often based on the belief that a contribution from the young can be obtained by means of research. That is to say, professional researchers make inventories of the wishes and needs of young people regarding provisions in their neighbourhoods; they systematically analyse these and convert them into recommendations for policy. The material thus obtained is then used to develop the policy, the idea being that in this way the young have been 'consulted'. Hazekamp (1993) classifies this modality under 'information' and in Hart's (1992) classification of participation levels (cf. page 37) this approach comes under step 5 of the ladder 'consulted and informed'. The characteristic is that the opinion of the young (for instance about urban renewal projects) has indeed been probed but that they were not involved in the analysis nor in possible policy decisions. A good example of this can be seen in the social renewal policy of the city of Rotterdam under the name Child in the City (KIDS). One part of the project, called Knee High Urban Renewal, is directed at increasing the liveability and practical value of the city for children. The aim is 'to take more account of children in the total design of outdoor spaces, not only by planning an (official) play area here and there, but by tuning the integral design to use by children' (Municipality of Rotterdam, 1991). Researchers were commissioned to study the use of space by children in three districts. This was intended to provide the answers to how children (and parents) value their neighbourhoods, which places they play in, how they get to these places, and what their wishes are for improvement. The study was carried out by means of interviews, questionnaires and observations. Now, without going into specific results, we come up against a fundamental question, namely what value can be ascribed to this way of collecting information. The approach has little to do with active participation; after all it only informs adults, and in particular policy-makers. One wonders why in such cases one-way traffic is chosen instead of two-way. Particularly in a situation in which changes in the living conditions and/or living environment of young people are concerned, it seems obvious to accord them an active role in the investigation process. It is quite possible to invite young people to participate instead of placing them in the passive position of data suppliers, leaving the power of interpretation entirely with the research workers and policy-makers. The children of the neighbourhood then join the research team as it were: 'together we are going to examine what is wrong with this neighbourhood, together we are going to see what solutions are conceivable and feasible, and together we are going to make every effort to get plans realized'. Depending on their ages, phase of development and abilities, young people – with guidance from specialists – can contribute to various stages of the investigation process. The contribution can consist, for instance, of group discussions on the questions put in the investigation, of conducting interviews, of simple categorization and/or formulation of conclusions and recommendations. In this way the character of the investigation becomes action-aimed[2]. From an educational point of view, the surplus value of such an approach is apparent. Not only is the balancing of supply and demand of provisions important, so is the fact that the young learn to put their own social needs into words, to respect the needs of others, and to weigh up differing interests and possibilities. In addition to these educational advantages, such an approach can yield profit on the research technical side, that is to say, in the validity[3] of the data obtained. van de Vall (1980, page 48) distinguishes two types of validity requirements that policy aimed investigations should meet: first the *'epistemological validity'* (the knowledge obtained must be an actual reflection of the current reality), and second the *'implemental validity'* (the knowledge must also be valid in relation to the policy that is intended to alter that reality). The involvement of children in the research process can promote both types of validity. A longer dialogue is started up in which the investigators can help children to word their opinions and needs as well as possible, and in which children in their turn can give the investigators a better insight into their motives. The experience that designers and youth workers have had in practice with children's participation in residential areas, shows time and time again that such a guiding process is necessary. If children are asked to make a design for a play area, they naturally react on the basis of the limited experience they possess at that moment. They chose what they already know about. New, creative ideas only arise after being confronted with other ideas and experiences, coming both from each other and from adults (Rijnen, 1989; Meindertsma, 1992). Such a dialogue is not necessary for younger children only. From the previously mentioned study by Hazekamp et al. (1993), it appears that older children do not feel that they are taken seriously unless they can easily communicate and discuss their project with adults. In other words, the value of information obtained from young people can increase if it evolves from a situation in which there is room for exchange of

---

[2]Action research is defined by van de Vall (1980, page 34) as 'investigation in which all those concerned in an organization or project field . . . themselves collect the data for the diagnosis, which are then passed to the organization to serve as a basis for new policy'.

[3]Validity is the degree to which a research procedure measures what it is supposed to measure.

experiences and confrontation with differing points of view. Not only does the reality value (epistemological validity) rise, but also the practical value with a view to the development of policy (implemental validity), because it is in this way that policy-makers obtain a considerably more mature final judgement from the young.

Hart (1992, pages 19 ff.) gives several good examples of such a participatory action research approach. The curricula of many British primary schools includes field studies, a type of project education strongly focused on the local neighbourhood and community. In this context, children carry out minor investigations of problems in their surroundings, for instance in the fields of housing, safety, traffic, places to play, etc. The results of such projects are invariably reported to the community and often to the local authority. In Hart's opinion, the great advantage of such an approach is that children obtain insight into the process of town planning and neighbourhood renewal. At the same time, the 'classic' subjects of geography, social studies and local history are stimulated because they can be combined with the tangible investigation experiences. Again in Britain, there are a number of Centres for Urban Studies where children and young people are given support, outside the educational framework, in carrying out studies of their surroundings. A well-known example is the Notting Dale Urban Studies Centre in West London. The institute provides instruction for the young researchers, helps them to formulate the research problems, supplies the necessary materials (tape recorders, photographic apparatus, etc.) and gives guidance in working out and analysing the results. All the research projects are put on file and are available to other groups of children, neighbourhood residents and policy-makers. In this way the Centre has become an information and support base for community participation. A previously mentioned Council of Europe Report (1993, cf. page 26) contains a description of a specific technique applied in countries including Germany, Norway and Sweden, for action research by young people. This is the Workbook Method, developed to involve neighbour-hood residents themselves in mapping out and solving problems in their surroundings. A group of the young set out in a workbook their ideas on a problem situation they themselves have recognized; the workbook is then distributed among groups of young people (and others involved). It is intended that these groups discuss the text and add their own analyses, suggestions and solutions. Thus a broader basis is created for activities that must eventually lead to resolving the problem. A recent Dutch example of research by the young is that of a study on the cultural orientation of schoolchildren in Amsterdam (Mudde, 1993). Guided by a research worker of the Free University, a group of five girls and six boys between 15 and 20 years old carried out an interview project to plot the leisure-time wishes and needs of the young in their own age group. The research was commissioned by a foundation that provides socio–cultural programmes for the young. A 'young-researcher's method' was chosen in order to keep the investigation 'as close as possible to the life-world of the target group'. Moreover, such a method matched the aims of the foundation. i.e. 'the cultural activation of boys and girls in order to increase their social participation and mobility' (ibid., page 7). The young who were interviewed indicated that they really appreciated being questioned by people of their own age. 'It gives you more confidence', 'it's easier to talk', and 'great, better than some old phoney' were some of their reactions (page 18). The young researchers were very enthusiastic too; the active participation gave them a sense of importance (page 67). It is not clear from the project report precisely what the foundation did with the results, and it is also hard to say whether this can be considered to be participatory action research in the sense described above.

In summary: children and young people as objects of research may produce useful information for policy development at local level, yet at the same time the process is so one-sided that it sidetracks the target group more than is necessary. It is precisely if changes in the direct residential environment are concerned that it is important to involve young people in the process. There young researchers can be excellent helpers. Not only do children learn a lot in the way of knowledge and skills, they are also being educated for citizenship. By participating in the investigation the young obtain experience of democratic processes at a local level and they learn the possibilities (and limitations) of their own active contribution. And finally the 'doing research together' will produce data that give more insight into the young's perception of the world, so increasing the relevance for the development of policy.

Conclusions

In recent years, local youth policy has been paying more attention to active commitment by children and young people. Three reasons can be indicated for this development. In the first place the youth itself is changing; the general social processes of democratization and emancipation that have taken place in the last decades have not left the young untouched. They stand up for their own opinions sooner, by no means always accept policy measures as self evident, and are less hesitant to resist matters which do not suit them. In the second place the attitude of policy-makers, administrators and professionals towards the young is changing. Whereas of old, youth policy had a strongly paternalistic character mainly aimed at 'uplifting' and in particular restraining the young, gradually more recognition has come for the contribution and capacities of this section of the population. This attitude is partly inspired by the assumption that the participation of young people may be an adequate manner to facilitate their social adjustment and fitting in (a reactive position). Yet there are also indications that a paradigmatic shift is taking place in local youth policy. Participation is being approached from a positive perspective, focused on the future. This vision can for instance be discerned within the socio-cultural child and youth work in which the dialogue with the young is seen more and more as a constituent of education and social education (Hazekamp *et al.*, 1994, page 115). In the third place a number of socio-economic factors are smoothing the path as it were for the participation of children and young people at the local level. One of the things we mentioned in this connection was the necessity felt by local authorities and housing associations to take more account, in a competitive market, of the changing wishes of the 'housing consumer'. Child-friendly surroundings proved to be an increasingly decisive factor here. In this sense, children's participation has a very practical function. It is a method to enhance the liveability of town and neighbourhood, and it thereby directly serves both financial and political interests.

If we look upon local youth policy in its entirety as socio-pedagogical practice, then the advancement of children's and youth participation emerges as a logical consequence. At the beginning of this chapter, we posited that every policy measure or intervention that relates to children will always influence their attitude towards society. Pursuing policy for, but over the heads of children creates distance that is in principle quite unnecessary. Not involving young people is also socially educative. It is a type of social education that contributes to the much-criticized figure of the irresponsible, calculating citizen who only pursues an individual interest and sees 'the government' as an anonymous, collective lucky dip. From this educational perspective, such an attitude towards citizenship can no longer be considered just a characteristic of individuals or, some believe, as a sign of the decline, originating in the family, of standards and values. It is also an attitude which was at least fostered by the way in which young people from childhood on were addressed by authorities and organizations. A municipal policy culture in which participation plays no role of any consequence, educates to immaturity, dependency or aggression. A policy that regularly invites the young to participate, conversely, promotes an attitude of social commitment, for today and tomorrow.

Naturally this is not to say that a local authority must make sure to hear the voice of youth for every trifle. The stimulation of participation in local youth policy means that the responsible adults accept entering into a dialogue with the young as a basic attitude, just as increasingly happens, for instance, in the case of designing neighbourhood environments. But a serious dialogue also implies that adults do not have to conceal their own knowledge, experience and opinions. The opinions of children and young people are, after all, formed to a great extent in confrontation with those of others, in particular of adults. The attitude towards the young is very clearly reflected in the way in which research regarding local youth policy is shaped. Here too, those who bear this responsibility should realize that the choice between research *about*, or research *with* the young has socio-pedagogical implications. Active participation of children and young people in research on their own surroundings is a very promising, but as yet underdeveloped means to education for citizenship.

References

ANACEJ (1992) *L'avenir citoyen*. Parijs: Assocation Nationale des Conseils d'Enfants et de Jeunes.

Bertels WPJ, JL Hazekamp & PH Kwakkelstein (1989) *De toekomst van gemeentelijk jeugdbeleid, deel I*. 's-Gravenhage: Vereniging van Nederlandse Gemeenten.

Bleeker H & K Mulderij (1982) *Kinderen wonen ook. Suggesties ter verbetering van een kindvergeten woonomgeving*. Deventer: Van Loghum Slaterus.

Bleeker H & K Mulderij (1984) *Pedagogiek op je knieën. Aspecten van kwalitatief-pedagogisch onderzoek*. Meppel: Boom.

Council of Europe (1993) *The development of an integrated approach to youth policy planning at local level*. Strasbourg: European Steering Committee for Intergovernmental Co-Operation in the Youth Field (CDEJ).

Faber J (1987) *Opvoeden in een pluriforme samenleving: over de samenhang van pedagogiek en recht*. Kampen: Kok Agora.

Hart RA (1992) *Children's participation. From tokenism to citizenship*. Florence, UNICEF Innocenti Essays nr. 4.

Hazekamp JL, J van der Gauw & J Nuijens (1993) *Jongeren doen mee aan beleid. Verslag van een onderzoek naar politieke participatie van jongeren op lokaal niveau*. 's-Gravenhage: VNG.

Hazekamp, JL, VA Leenders, MAC Valkestijn & DJR Verwer (1994) *Sociaal-cultureel jeugdwerk. Stand van zaken en perspectieven*. Utrecht: NIZW.

Imelman JD (1974) *Plaats en inhoud van een personale pedagogiek. Een bijdrage tot begripsanalytisch en fenomenologisch denken*. Dissertatie RU Groningen. Groningen: Wolters-Noordhof.

Langeveld MJ ea (1952) *Maatschappelijke verwildering der jeugd. Rapport betreffende het onderzoek naar de geestesgesteldheid van de massajeugd*. 's-Gravenhage: Staatsuitgeverij.

Meindertsma SW (1992) *Presentatie kinderinspraakprojecten*. Studiebijeenkomst Raad voor het Jeugdbeleid, 10-11-1992.

Mudde S (1993) *Het is saai als het de hele tijd hetzelfde is. Een onderzoek naar de culturele oriëntatie van jongens en meisjes in de vrije tijd.* Amsterdam: Stichting Arena

NUSO (1984) *Kinderinspraak.* Interne uitgave. Amsterdam: NUSO.

NUSO (1993) *Het speelruimteweb. Het speelruimteplan als deel van de gemeentelijke planologie.* Utrecht: NUSO.

Rijnen J (1989) *Vraag het ze zelf. Praktijkboek kinderinspraak bij het inrichten van speelruimte.* Utrecht: LANS.

Salman HHA (1993) Lezing studiedag '*Begeleiding van kinderinspraak-projecten*' Landelijk Kinderwerkoverleg. Utrecht, 8-6-1993.

Sturkenboom FCH (1993) *Kinderen in de volkshuisvesting.* Lezing NUSO-congres 'Spelen is een kunst'; Laren, 17-6-1993. Utrecht: NUSO (interne uitgave).

Vall M van de (1980) *Sociaal beleidsonderzoek. Een professioneel paradigma.* Alphen ad Rijn: Samsom.

Visser F (1993) *Girafglijbaan met uitkijktoren.* Amsterdam: Raad voor het Jeugdbeleid.

Participation in education

Education is treated as a means of acquiring power over the pupil, not as a means of nourishing his own growth. Among children the joy of mental adventure is far commoner than in grown men and women. It is rare in later life because everything is done to kill it during education... Education should not aim at a passive awareness of dead facts but at an activity directed towards the world that our efforts are to create. It should be inspired, not by a regretful hankering after the extinct beauties of Greece and the Renaissance, but by a shining vision of the society that is to be, of the triumphs that thought will achieve in the time to come... All through education, initiative should come from the pupil as far as possible... Those who are taught in this spirit will be filled with life and hope and joy, able to bear their part in bringing to mankind a future less sombre than the past, with faith in the glory that human effort can create...'

(Bertrand Russell, 1916)[1]

Introduction

And what about schools? If there is any educational environment which sets out, at least verbally, to give young people forward-looking education for citizenship, it is school. 'In most of today's educational programmes', says educationalist Deen (1992), 'we encounter a pursuit of the pupil's independence and autonomy. But in practice this ideal looks very much like remaining an abstraction'. In general pupils 'are not taken seriously as human beings and find themselves still subjected to a process of education for obedience and tutelage'. According to Deen, today's school sends out a double message. The slogans proclaiming pupils' own responsibility and autonomy are not followed up in day-to-day reality: democracy within the school organization is practically non-existent, possibilities to function independently and the right to participate in decision-making are found only sporadically. What was said in the previous chapter on local youth policy, namely that the way it deals with young people by definition offers them a major learning experience as to how they are appreciated as citizens, applies to an even greater degree to the educational system. After all the school itself is in two respects an experience of penetrating education for

---

[1]From: Bertrand Russell on Education, in Rubenstein & Stoneman (1970).

citizenship. Firstly it is an institution, a social organization in which children spend a major part of their youth. As well as absorbing cognitive subject matter they gain considerable experience of the manner in which adults deal with each other and with children, of how in society people are ordered in relation to one another, in other words, of civil values such as democratic outlook, respect, responsibility, plurality and solidarity. If a serious dialogue is held with the children at school about the school itself, for instance by discussing the content, organization and criteria of education with them, they learn that their opinion and commitment is appreciated and that their contribution is respected. Where such a dialogue is lacking and own initiatives are discouraged rather than stimulated, the implicit lesson is: citizenship is fine, but not under my roof! In present-day education however, the latter practice dominates by far (Deen, 1992; Diekstra, 1992). Secondly, the school provides vital practice in citizenship, because it usually plays a major part within a local community. Primary school in particular is often a neighbourhood facility, which in principle offers many opportunities to practise actual social participation. In the previous chapter we gave the example of the commitment of primary school pupils to neighbourhood projects on play areas and traffic safety. In this way not only cognitive competencies are learned, but civic values are also generated. The opportunities for social participation starting from schools are only very occasionally used, however.

Of old, education for citizenship has been a major theme in discussions on educational reform. Educationalists such as Kohnstamm and Langeveld considered education for citizenship to be a major aim of education. In this connection they advocated didactic methods that took 'learning to learn' and 'learning to think' as their starting points. It is on their work that the present argument is based for 'developmental education', in which 'pupils are brought to ever greater independent action through self-motivation' (Carpay, 1994). In the context of education for citizenship many educational reformers, such as Dewey, Freinet and Boeke conducted experiments in school democratization. In the present period as well, initiatives are taken in this direction, for example in the shape of representative advisory councils and the pupils' charter. However, public discussion on education has always been characterized by movements which firmly rejected such a development on grounds of principle. The psychologist Hofstee maintains that in regard to citizenship the educational system should restrict itself to the teaching of the essential cognitive skills, for instance in the shape of 'social science' (Hofstee, 1992). In this way he refers to the teaching of a number of 'proven' social-psychological and political facts, as well as 'a range of procedures humankind has thought up to control social processes such as the commission, the delegation, the dispensation, the civil office and so on'. Hofstee resolutely rejects as indoctrination all other activities conceivable with respect to education for citizenship at school, because they would involve a 'moral component which affects the pupil's integrity and perverts the very fibre of education'.

By definition, education, like local youth policy, is an educational context for citizenship. Whether the school handles relevant activities as an explicit part of the curriculum, or to the contrary takes pains to avoid them, it always presents the children with a picture of society and their position within it. Because this process of socialization is inevitable it is even more important to closely examine shape and content of the process, as well as its possible effects. In the first place, via a brief historical survey, we shall have a closer look at the various points of view as to the task of the educational system with respect to citizenship. Such points of view are not, of course, isolated phenomena, but are emphatically connected with broad developments in society and specifically with the view taken of the relationship between society and the school. Subsequently we examine to what extent present education shapes the pupils' social commitment and participation. In this connection the social climate in the school itself is important, but also the way in which and the extent to which the school is oriented towards society. A separate section is devoted to the question of standards and values in education. This is a politically topical theme which reflects the anxiety many adults feel about the behaviour of 'the young'. However, it is interesting, in the light of the social commitment of young people, to see how the subject is handled within the education system. A major question is whether standards and values can be learned within the school in an abstract manner (through representation), without the school itself in its organization setting the example, and so providing opportunity for practice.

Citizenship in the education system

Making more people more competent (Meer mensen mondig maken) was the title of a booklet in which, in 1975, the Netherlands Ministry of Education and Science endeavoured to promote the 'contours of a future education system' (Ahlers, 1975). Reading or re-reading this 20-year-old manifesto one is impressed by at least two things: in the first place by the fact that the themes broached in it are still very topical, and secondly by the enormous optimism with regard to the possibilities of educational reform the text displays. The major principles of the policy proposed for educational reform were: combating the inequality in educational and thus career opportunities, broadening the school curriculum, and promoting consultation and participation in decision-making. All of these are subjects that play a prominent part in the current debate on education. It is precisely this point that proves how stubborn reforms in the field of education are.

The policy met with political resistance as well as the conservatism of the educational system itself. This shows that changes argued from the perspective of children and young people often remain plans as long as the time is not ripe. What are the past and present views on equal opportunities, content of education and the position of pupils?

Maintaining positions

Education is the mirror of society. For centuries formal education was a privilege for the children of the elite. People who were not of that class were prepared for later life at home or in the workshop. In medieval, feudal societies 'learning' for most lower-class children only meant being employed in family labour. Children of ordinary townspeople could be apprenticed, from the age of seven, to a Master of a Guild who would initiate them into the craft. Education in schools was in the hands of the Roman Catholic church. The latter deigned to make perfect only the children of the ruling classes, by teaching them, besides faith, also the principles of higher arts. Education was literally in the service of 'maintaining positions', because the station into which one was born constituted the main principle of ordering pre-modern society. After the Middle Ages vast social changes were set in motion. Trade and the products of craftsmanship increasingly determined the economic face of society, the feudal structure slowly gave way to an establishment in which the merchants of the cities held power. They proceeded to found their own schools. Subjects were Latin, the financial system and the law; these being deemed necessary for rising world trade. So-called reading and writing schools were founded for the children of craftsmen, who were taught mainly the vernacular and arithmetic. Education for the poor began to develop only as the Reformation manifested itself. The various denominations saw the school as a means to hold on to more believers, and to lessen the financial burden of poor relief. This education had little substance. In crowded premises underpaid schoolmasters confined themselves to instruction in biblical knowledge, discipline and order. This picture hardly changed until the beginning of the nineteenth century. The well-to-do citizens met their needs with Latin (later French) schools. Popular education was mainly a form of poor relief in which the leading motive was discipline. Within the new bourgeois society the major aim of education was still maintaining positions.

From the nineteenth century the rise of nationalism in Europe gave new meaning to education. Around 1800 the Netherlands developed into a unified state, in strong competition with other states. Socialization to citizenship, patriotism and discipline by means of a national system of education was to become the cement of this building of a new nation. Free popular education was introduced, the central elements of which were standard Dutch, national history and geography. This Dutch popular education had little to do with the contemporary ideals which were characteristic of the French Revolution: liberty, equality and fraternity. The liberal bourgeoisie on the contrary was greatly worried by the danger of the education system undermining ordinary people's class consciousness. Roland Holst (Dutch poet and socialist) cites (1902) a worried member of the board of the Municipal Schools for the Poor as saying:

> *In order to safeguard you, who are affluent, the schools for the poor, which are ours and yours and which are training grounds for duty and order, should be promoted, maintained, assisted and supported. The poor must learn to read so as to be able to understand your will, know their duty, follow the rules for good behaviour and learn good and improving hymns. The only science in which they are instructed is the doctrine of their dependence and servitude: it is the aptitude to live in orderliness and quietitude and to be of use to their fellow-citizens, country and monarch: it is that each should know his place in society...*

Though not all children by far were reached by this popular education, and though it had little substance as yet, in an unexpected way it was the occasion for the gradual generalization of school attendance. The liberal initiatives in this field in fact provoked strong reactions from denominational groups, who felt their 'market position' was under threat. Roman Catholics and Protestants were equally afraid of the secularizing influence state education might have on the population. The resulting controversy on school funding stimulated school attendance in two ways. The provision of education was increased because in the competitive struggle denominational and state schools, as well as non-denominational private schools, were founded everywhere, and the demand for education was strengthened because the various elites more and more coerced their clients to attend their schools (de Vries, 1993, page 29). When finally, around 1900, compulsory education was introduced, most children had been going to school for a long time already, busy becoming civilized and superior. Diligence, neatness and obedience after all were generally accepted to be essential values. The bourgeois elites saw this school attendance as an important means to counteract social unrest resulting from poverty and unemployment, and to meet the need for disciplined labour. For the working classes themselves education was a means to raise social mobility. The civilizing offensive of the bourgeoisie and the pursuit of emancipation of the lower classes appeared to go hand in hand. Nevertheless the social stratification of education remained largely unaffected. Vocational training came into being for working class children, such as the technical school for boys and domestic subjects for girls. Children from the bourgeoisie went to

Gymnasium and Hogere Burgerschool (secondary schools with an emphasis on either classical languages or on subjects more suitable to trade and industry).

Although social mixing happened on a moderate scale only, there were possibilities for it in principle. The exceptional cases in which this succeeded (the child of a skilled labourer who via secondary modern and teachers' training college managed to become a teacher) confirmed the belief in the unprecedented opportunities offered by education to the talented who were willing to exert themselves. de Vries (1993, page 70) calls this the 'meritocratic idea: the ideology which says that social role assignment takes place on grounds of achieved status and not, as in the class society, on grounds of ascribed status'. For that matter, according to this author, a 'lucky catch' status is often hidden behind the achieved status. Within this ideological context, inequality in education and society was for a long time accepted as fact. The insight that specific, often hidden selection mechanisms in school played a major part in maintaining this stratification was recognized only long after the Second World War, and then by no means by everybody.

Equal opportunities

As stated above, in about 1975 the Dutch authorities found that children from a working class environment had considerably less opportunity to move on to higher types of education than children from the higher classes, and that for girls, opportunities in education as well as for a career in society were considerably smaller than for boys. Children of parents with little education still leave school with lower marks and less prestigious certificates than children from the middle classes (Bakker *et al.*, 1993, page 68). The disadvantage is particularly great for children from ethnic minorities (ABOP, 1989; Kerkhoff, 1989). The emancipation policy for education so far has yielded insufficient results, especially for Turkish and Moroccan girls. Apparently the education system is hard put to breach or even slightly modify social inequality on the basis of socio-cultural and socio-economic backgrounds. Sometimes the educational system is thought to have the explicit effect of reproducing and increasing inequality. de Vries (1993) mentions two causes. Because all children are obliged to go to school (compulsory education), education becomes the central distributor of social opportunities. The certificate obtained largely decides the place pupils will later occupy in the social pecking order. These certificates, however, are subject to heavy inflation. The qualifications obtained as well as the educational requirements are constantly stepped up. In this way education retains its meritocratic character. Early in life children already have to come to terms with the idea that in school as well as in society 'might is right' applies. Clearly, this right is not based on talent, intelligence and ability only. Since they obtain a 'surplus of cultural capital' at home, children from the higher classes appear to profit much more from the education offered than other children (ibid., page 75).

One of the most poignant examples illustrating this harsh selection process is the referral or expulsion of ever more children from regular education to special schools. This type of education, originally meant as an educational safety net for children with learning problems, has grown by two to three thousand pupils per year since the 1960s, notwithstanding the fall in the total number of births (Doornbos, 1991). Since research shows that this constant increase cannot be explained by some sort of epidemic of learning disorders, so-called 'system effects' should obviously be looked for: mechanisms in education and society which stimulate this expulsion. Doornbos mentions as the main factors: the pressure from society on education (higher standards, higher expectations from parents, stricter testing of study results due to an increasing achievement mentality), competition between schools in a shrinking market for pupils, and the conflict of interests between various sectors and professions. All this results in a systematic 'casting out of unfit children' from regular education, wrapped up in an argument in which the interests of all parties seems to be served (ibid., page 25). The children concerned are looked after better, with a focus on their individual needs. The other pupils and the teacher are not 'held up', and the referring school maintains its level of performance and good name. Since the 1970s several attempts have been made to stem this trend, on the basis of educational as well as financial motives. The most recent plan is 'Weer Samen naar School' (Together to School Again). The ultimate goal of the plan is to take care of as many children with learning problems as possible within regular education (Ministry of Education and Science, 1990). The prospects for actually realizing this plan however are not altogether favourable[2]. In the meantime special education continues to grow, and with it 'apartheid' in the Dutch educational system (Doornbos, 1991). In this way children are made familiar at an early age with the 'circumstance' that there are suitable and unsuitable citizens. They are told that this selection takes place on the basis of individual talent and merit, and not, as used to be the case explicitly, on the basis of class or birth. This implicit lesson in citizenship, that is to say in the manner in which schools produce and reproduce inequalities between different groups of citizens, undoubtedly has a far-reaching influence on the pupils' development and self-image. There is after all no reason to underestimate the power of

---

[2]The major preconditions for implementation, as formulated by the author of the plan, which include bringing down the size of groups to 24 pupils and an increase of teaching staff of primary schools, do not look politically practicable (Doornbos, 1994; de Graaff, 1994).

observation of children and young people. Day in, day out, they experience how the system, for example through the assessment of their cognitive achievements, pre-selects them for what Doornbos calls the social tripartition into ordinary citizens, second-class citizens and first-class citizens. Most children who fall by the wayside, moreover, learn to accept their individual lot willingly, and are even grateful. Most of them after all have had extremely unpleasant experiences of continuous failure and inadequacy, which is why the extra care and attention they receive in the special schools must be a relief. The price they ultimately have to pay for their early dropping out will be apparent only after they have left school[3].

Nature and content of the education process

Schooling, the introduction of young people into culture and society, has in Deen's opinion (1992, pages 94 ff.), three dimensions as to content, namely *instrumentation, orientation* and *community building*. Instrumentation comprises the basic techniques for the acquisition of knowledge, such as reading, writing, arithmetic, verbalization, use of resources etc. Orientation refers to the cultural content of what is learned, in other words the presentation and acquisition of knowledge about various domains of spiritual and social life. Community building is the socialization process; familiarizing children with life in a larger framework. In present-day schools the first two dimensions are explicitly encountered. The major part of the curriculum consists of subjects that are to equip the pupils cognitively for further education and work. These are heavily emphasized, because the quality of education is still measured mainly by the level of knowledge reached. Moreover, instrumentation is considered the hard core of education, because it can be taught in curriculum elements and can be assessed objectively. The dimension of orientation is mainly present in subjects such as civics or world orientation, religious knowledge and creative courses. These are the subjects which are at the heart of frequent dispute in educational circles. Only a few years after a number of these 'orientation elements' were introduced into Dutch primary education, they are now already under attack. Some consider orientation to be excess baggage, which is said to lower the level of education. Community building, to end up with, generally gets little attention. It could be said that this is manifested especially through the 'hidden curriculum', the standards

---

[3]The 'care by segregation' does not only operate through special schools. Doornbos (1991, pages 54 ff.) finds that many primary schools which have a surplus of pupils from socially weak groups and for that reason receive extra government facilities in the framework of the priority education policy, show great similarity in many respects with schools for special education. The social stratification is even more severe in secondary education.

and values which play a strongly regulating part in schools, but which usually remain implicit. We shall return to this later.

The problems of selection and segregation discussed in the previous section are, of course, closely related to the content of education. And in its turn the content cannot be considered separately from the demands made on education by society. Practically every parent wants his or her child to have the highest possible certificate in the assumption that it will give the best chance of a good social position. A certificate indeed has an important screening function. It informs a future employer or institute of further education not only about cognitive and/or technical skills, but also on the social skills which are needed to complete the course or hold down the job successfully. But what was once a valuable certificate is not necessarily so valuable now. In the previous section we already mentioned the inflation of these documents, and the ever higher demands made on young people. What does the certificate MAVO (lower general secondary education) yield in social perspective nowadays, and what opportunities does HAVO (upper general secondary education) still offer? As inflation and external requirements increase, children are 'compelled' to ever higher education. The fact that many schools have decided to introduce a test for failure anxiety for all pupils is therefore hardly surprising. In short, the Peter Principle seems to play a part in education. Pupils are pushed upwards (with the best of intentions), until a number of them have risen to the level of their incompetence, with all the psychosocial consequences.

The driving onward of pupils takes place particularly in the field of cognition, so in the orientation dimension. From the point of view of community building, however, other aspects than intellectual ones are important as well. Calling to mind the descriptions of the concept of citizenship given in Chapter 2, it is clear that quite a few demands are made on future citizens. van Gunsteren (1992) defines this citizen as someone who 'is capable of fulfilling the twin roles of governing and being governed in an autonomous, judicious and loyal way'. We shall not repeat the discussion on definitions here, but it is certainly clear that there is a lot to be learned and taught in this field. These capacities and attitudes after all do not just come naturally. The history of education shows that ruling elites as well as passionate reformers have always seen the social education of the young as one of the main aims of schooling. The content of that education and the precise aim one wanted to achieve depended and still depends by definition on political, ideological or philosophical ideas, in other words the way in which the future of society was, and still is, seen. As said before, until well into the nineteenth century education explicitly meant 'maintaining'. Children from the elites were prepared for the positions of power they were to inherit, and once the children of the 'rabble' went to school the intention was chiefly to make them true followers of the church, the monarch or the country. This did not involve many educational and social advantages. Their education was little more than training in discipline, coercion to willingly accept their position in the margin of society. The high ideals of the Enlightenment (cf. page 48) could change little in this respect. Schooling to educate children, through knowledge and civilization, to be free, rational individuals was for a long time solely available to the children of the emerging bourgeoisie. It was only under the influence of growing industrialization in the second half of the nineteenth century that it came to be considered profitable for popular education to be something more than pure training in discipline. The economy required literate labour, therefore the children from the working classes also had to be schooled – in the modern sense of the word. This is the moment, symbolized in the Netherlands by the introduction of general compulsory education, that may be considered the beginning of modern education. Now it held good for all children that school was to promote their intellectual and social capabilities and to educate them to 'Christian and social virtues'. The latter was a formula which had already been laid down in the Primary Education Act of 1857, in the thick of the school funding controversy[4].

Reforms

Although from that time onwards education has been available for everybody, children were still hardly taken into account. Schools were organized on the basis of age, in classes with large numbers of children, the major goal being to inculcate fixed subject matter and rules of behaviour. If only for physical reasons, individual differences between children could scarcely be taken into account. Moreover, children's individual interests were not part of the vocabulary of school and society. Until well into this century fashioning children into useful, that is economically profitable and socially well-adjusted, individuals remained the dominant educational practice. It was this very denial of the distinct nature of the individual, that was targeted by a reform movement, which arose in the course of the nineteenth century: *Reform pedagogy*[5]. German philosophers and educationalists in particular turned away from what they felt to be the extremely mechanistic, materialist and rationalist image of man which had emerged under the influence of industrialization. They deemed this development a

---

[4]The class character of schools, however, did not disappear with the introduction of compulsory education. Officially the classification of schools according to the level of fees was prohibited, but the founding of schools outside the state system was increasingly used as a covert way to provide separate education for children of the well-to-do.

[5]For a fuller description see *inter alia* Teunissen (1992).

denial of the natural character of man, and they saw children in particular as a source of change. The education system was a major object of this movement. In Chapter 2 some educational experiments, set up in this light, were reviewed. The reform educationalists in the first place wanted more notice to be taken of the child's distinct nature. The aim of education should be the full development of individual talent and potential. The period of youth was considered a phase of life with its own meaning, not to be measured by the dominant standard of adult culture. School should base itself on the unique development every child goes through, taking into account each child's talents, possibilities and needs. In the place of 'fixed subject matter' the children were to be offered 'the material for learning'.

The ideas of these reformers constituted a radical break with existing thinking in education. But they did not gain a decisive influence; apparently the time was not yet ripe. What was put into practice was the founding of a few progressive schools, based for instance on the principles of Montessori, Dalton or Decroly. A number of representatives of Reform pedagogy also linked individualized education to a social objective. Not only was the school to be a safe youthland in which childhood could blossom freely, the school should also educate for democratic functioning within the 'new society'. The American educationalist Dewey, around the turn of the century, advocated an entirely different organization and content for schooling, by which the gap between abstract knowledge and physical and social reality was to be closed. This gap, according to Dewey, had arisen mainly through industrialization, which had caused a separation of learning and experience. In *The school and society* (1899) and *Democracy and education* (1923) he stated his philosophy of learning by doing. School should be a social working community where children as young scientists experiment with natural objects and production techniques, enabling them in this way to visualize the development of knowledge that mankind has experienced. Not before they themselves, in cooperation with each other, have been able to gain the experience of the evolution of knowledge and have learnt in stages to apply it, will a positive, progress-oriented attitude of learning and living ensue. Dewey held the opinion that authoritarian relations do not fit into such a social laboratory situation. A democratic, fast-changing society can function only when its members have learned to take their own initiatives and adapt to new circumstances. 'Otherwise, they will be overwhelmed by changes in which they are caught and whose significance or connections they do not perceive. The result will be a confusion in which a few will appropriate to themselves the results of the blind and externally directed activities of others' (1923, pages 101,102). School can only actually contribute to education for democracy if it manages to challenge children to mutual interest, to active commitment to one another's work and to mutual communication. Comparable ideas were at the root of the Workshop Children's Community, founded in 1926 (Kuipers, 1992). In this Dutch school too self-motivation and self-development were at the centre; here also the emphasis was on integration of learning and doing. Community education by 'sociocracy' was taken extremely seriously. In weekly discussions decisions were only made if all those present, including therefore all children aged from 3 to 18, could agree. After the Second World War the radical character of this educational experiment was soon lost, mainly because the school had financial problems that forced it to apply for state funding. It had to conform to state requirements such as group teaching, a 'normal' curriculum and recognized final examinations.

Although at that time the influence of these reform movements was fairly restricted, they have set the tone for the educationalist debate going on to the present day. Considering afresh the Dutch policy for educational reform in the mid-1970s, we see again the criticism of the education system that clearly shows the marks of Reform pedagogy:

> *Present-day education dates back to a time when the premise was that the pupil had to be taught as much knowledge as possible. We now understand that by this one-sided approach education has neglected quite a number of tasks. Pupils for instance obtain insufficient insight into the society they live in. Mastery of the subject matter is often still considered a goal in itself and not a means to get a grip on reality. The split-up into specialized subjects often makes it hard for pupils to see larger contexts. Moreover education insufficiently stimulates pupils to self-motivation, to make a contribution and to take their own stand. In this way many pupils will later still not be competent but socially vulnerable. Not because they have learned nothing at school, but because they have not learned sufficiently to apply the knowledge. Education is mainly targeted at the development of rational and technical qualities. In particular in secondary and higher education, but also in elementary education very little attention is paid to physical education, to articulateness, to artistic education or to the development of the emotional life ... All this has led to a stunting of personal development, ... and for that reason more attention will have to be paid to creative arts, to individualization and mutual cooperation.*
>
> *(Ahlers, 1975, page 15)*

Consequently a broadening of the educational curriculum was advocated for all children up to 16 years old, in the shape of a standardized foundation: the primary school and the comprehensive school. In regard to the new primary school, now including 4- and 5-year-olds, this aim has been realized for the greater part. The Primary Education Act of 1985 states *inter alia* that 'education will be organized in such a way as to enable pupils to pass through an uninterrupted development process' and education will 'in any case be directed at emotional and intellectual development, and at the development of creativity, at the acquisition of the necessary knowledge and social, cultural and physical skills'. The proposals for a comprehensive school were less successful. The political opposition as well as the resistance in secondary education circles against this type of education, dubbed 'boringly uniform', was so strong that it never got beyond a few experiments. The idea behind the comprehensive school – extended basic education for all pupils to provide them with a broadened and standardized foundation for further education and the labour market – was the model, in a cut-down version, for the 'basic education' introduced into secondary education in 1993. Since then, care, technology and information science have been included with the traditional subjects in the core curriculum for all 12- to 16-year-olds.

The content of the educational curriculum has unmistakably been broadened in the last few years. Pupils' 'personality development' has become more central, more attention is being paid to orientation subjects and individual guidance, and self-motivation is increasingly stimulated. These are elements which not only make life at school more pleasant, they are important conditions from a perspective of education for citizenship as well. 'How amused people were about care as a school subject', says a member of a national commission which had to supervise the introduction of basic education. 'But it really stands for more than learning how to clean your teeth. In the end it is about your care of yourself, about taking responsibility in a broad sense, so that you may become a constructive member of society' (Schöttelndreier, 1994). The question however is to what extent the latter aim can be given concrete form within the present organization of education. To actually teach pupils how to carry social responsibility and to feel committed to what happens in society around them, 'becoming acquainted with' and 'talking about', however important, is not enough. A further 'socialization' of the school is needed, in two respects. In the first place an opportunity must be created within education to practise this social responsibility. In the second place an open connection should come into being between school and society. Education for citizenship, in the sense of community education, can evolve only through continuous interaction of abstract theories and actual practice.

Community education, standards and values

Should in fact schools educate children to become democratic citizens; is that their task? As said before, opinions are divided on this issue. The reports of the Dutch Scientific Advisory Board on Government Policy (WRR) on *Citizenship in our time* (see Chapter 2) take up an ambivalent position (WRR, 1992a,b,c). 'A theory of citizenship which concentrates on, or expects any good from, upbringing or education is suspect for that very reason' they state. 'What adult citizens cannot at the moment achieve amongst themselves is passed on to the educators (themselves adult citizens) and the children. At best this is investing in the future, but irresponsible wishful thinking usually lies at the bottom of that too... Education and upbringing must not be used to solve problems of citizenship. They should give access to existing citizenship – no more and no less' (van Gunsteren, 1992, page 7). Then again there are phrases in, for instance, the Primary Education Act and the Act on Basic Education, which do indeed mention socio-cultural education as core objectives of the curriculum. Current discussions and policy intentions around the educational assignment of school by definition relate to community education.

However this may occur, education hands children an apparatus of knowledge, skills and attitudes which structures their image of mankind and society to a considerable extent. Social knowledge, to which the psychologist Hofstee wants to restrict community education in schools, looks on the face of it like non-normative, impartial interpretation. But the 'enculteration' at school naturally does not confine itself to a designated set of lessons or study module. And, certainly in its applications, knowledge is never entirely free from values. Besides that, the hidden curriculum is chock-full of social values and standards. These express themselves for example in the appreciation of various capabilities, in the way teachers and pupils associate, in the way in which the school is organized, and in the way in which social phenomena are discussed. In short: community education takes place through instruction and orientation, but either explicitly or implicitly also through the social climate at school. Therefore whether or not this education is the task of the school is not very relevant.

According to educationalist Lea Dasberg (1993), the educational system has, in the course of time, equipped itself with numerous rationalizations to keep education (both individual and social) out and restrict itself to socialization. The latter concept she defines as 'introducing the child into the given society', and is therefore of a conformist character. Education however, for her is a moral assignment. It implies that children are taught to have a critical attitude towards the world around them, so as to be able to develop their own (social) ideal for the future. Some of these rationalizations have been mentioned before: education in this sense would amount to indoctrination, and education is not a task of the school but of the family. Besides this it is often argued that the heterogeneity of the group of pupils does not allow schools to take up a prescriptive or ideological position[6]. Dasberg however does not consider the pluralistic character of

---

[6]The educationalist JD Imelman takes up a comparable relativist position, when he observes that 'there are hardly any universally manageable standards and values left'. 'Searching for them in this time of transborder communication is nostalgically harking back to the orderly nineteenth century' (Volkskrant, November 10, 1993).

society a reason to refrain from moral education at school: 'this argument may be refuted by pointing out that the standards and values of democracy are, consciously or unconsciously, accepted by practically every citizen and need not make any home front of the pupils feel threatened' (ibid., page 6). A last important reason for advocating a separation of schooling and education is to be found, according to Dasberg, in the adults' crisis of values. If adults themselves have difficulty painting their picture of the future, if they themselves have serious doubts about the cultural and social content they are to transfer, moral education looks like a very hazardous venture indeed[7].

The question poses itself whether it is at all possible to phrase an aim as to content for community education or moral development that does not in advance fall victim to ideological warfare. Dasberg is of the opinion that moral education does not equal telling the pupils what is good and what is bad. According to her, moral education means that pupils are acquainted with the 'problem of morality, without supplying ready-made solutions' (ibid., pages 16,17). To arrive at one's position by discussion: this builds the conscience of responsible, critical spirits. With that intention various programmes have been designed which target either 'values clarification' or the promotion of cognitive development. The values clarification programme, introduced by the American researchers Raths and Simon (1975), takes as its point of departure that children should learn to choose their values themselves from various possible alternatives. They have to argue as best they can the choice they make in the lesson and are subsequently encouraged to act according to the values chosen. Absolute neutrality of the teachers is essential. The authors require them to avoid any directive suggestions and restrict themselves to offering possibilities for the children to make their own choices. This approach entails various problems. Firstly, much research shows that it just does not work. From a literature study by Lockwood (1978) it appears that neither the values themselves, nor the consciousness of them are substantially influenced. Moreover, the programmes proved to have hardly any of the tangible behavioural effect that was intended. Even more serious are the findings of Damon (1988), who shows that the value–neutrality propagated has the opposite effect: such a position induces the pupils to passive indifference and cynicism with regard to moral choices. 'Why should a child bother working through a moral problem, or risk taking a stand, when a child's supposed moral mentor refrains from doing so?' is how Damon explains this attitude (pages 149,150). The programmes intended to stimulate the children's cognitive development level require the teacher to take up a clear

---

[7]The educationalist Mollenhauer (1986, pages 18, 19) speaks in the same vein, saying that education makes no sense if adults no longer know whether or not their values and standards are worth passing on to their children.

position. These methods, based on the theories of Kohlberg (cf. page 64), depart from the conviction that children during their process of development acquire ever higher moral positions. From this perspective it is the teacher's task to further the moral growth, to point out the shortcomings or inconsistencies in their reasoning, and to confront them with 'basic values' such as honesty, justice, solidarity and democratic attitudes (Kohlberg, 1970; Damon, 1988). Lockwood's previously mentioned literature study shows that such an approach to discussion does have an effect: the method proves to be capable of significantly raising the level of moral argument.

The two techniques for instruction in standards and values have a common fault however, namely that moral reasoning is conceived as an isolated activity. Kohlberg himself argued for embedding his moral development programme in an educational system which was to be organized on the principles of a participatory democracy[8], so that pupils could learn actually to apply the knowledge obtained. However, his method too is generally taught as an isolated classroom activity. Usually the 'morality' lessons are detached from the other subjects at school, and from the actual practice confronting children inside as well as outside school. Thus it may be the case that through Kohlberg's technique children attain the highest level of moral reasoning ('justice' and 'democratic attitudes'), yet experience the opposite in the day-to-day practice at school. What is concerned here, as Deen states, is a psychological approach to the theory of values separating practice and morality (1992, page 73). We find the same psychological approach in the political argument around the strengthening of values and standards and the educational assignment of the school. Fearing what in the first half of the century was called 'the unruliness of mass youth', and now reads 'a threatening drop-out of marginalized young people', politicians seek refuge in an old remedy, namely to have the school act as a master of morals. This remedy did not work in the past because the level of the intervention was not correct. The working class children, then the target group, were not much impressed because there was a huge gap between the morals preached and their actual conditions of life. Probably it will not work now either, because the connection between theory and practice is lacking. A group of young people in a morals lesson discussing the problems of refugees and asylum seekers, and the question whether the country is 'full', are challenged, as it were, to take up non-committal standpoints, even if the teacher does his very best to set 'basic values' against them. For some pupils, opinion forming will move into an idealistic or socially desirable direction, others will feel the need to react against it and shout racist slogans.

---

[8]Kohlberg (1985) uses the term 'just community school'.

Moral development is closely connected with the social experience children gradually obtain. Painstaking studies by Damon (1979, 1988) into social and moral development prove that morality increases in 'natural social interaction'. Social commitment does not, according to him, evolve from the confrontation with ideas, but from the actual experiences the child acquires in his day-to-day relationships: 'If we want to train passive subjects of a totalitarian state, we should be careful to provide children only with relationships in which they are mindless recipients of indoctrination. If, on the other hand, we want democratic citizens, we should provide for them relationships in which they can think, argue, and freely make choices' (1988, page 146). Damon therefore argues for a link between moral education in the classroom and practical experience in and out of school. By applying this understanding to the example of refugees we gave above, a different situation arises. The class might visit a reception centre for refugees, and talk direct to fellow youngsters about their experiences of war and terrorism. Moral dilemmas become real when refugees tell their story, and put the question to the pupils: 'wouldn't you yourself have fled in such a situation?', or 'how would you feel if you were a refugee and not welcome anywhere?' A non-committal attitude is less likely in such direct confrontation. Any statement or opinion produces its direct, visible consequences. A pupil who wants to insist that the country is overcrowded would have to tell the young refugee: 'as far as I am concerned, you will have to go back to the country where you were tortured'. This is much less easy than 'tough talking' in a lesson on clarification of values. A somewhat more light-hearted example: within a didactic method like Rath's, a certain value is put up for discussion, for instance 'obedience'. The question is what are its limits: should one obey rules one has not been consulted about or which one absolutely disagrees with? Children are now encouraged to take up a position, consider alternatives and consequences, put their opinion into words in the group, and subsequently act according to this opinion. They may, after serious consultation, have arrived at the conclusion that one should stick to rules which, with everybody's consent, were agreed upon in the interest of the whole group. In that case they have a right to expect the school organization to act in accordance. If the latter does not do so – a teacher at the start of the year sets the rules for everybody to obey – then a start is made on undermining a democratic morality which is precisely what people often say they want to promote.

In modern education children are continually placed in this type of double bind. Deen in this connection points at the phenomenon of cooperation: 'on the one hand lip service is paid to the importance of cooperation, whereas as soon as children try to put it into practice (as they see it), helping each other is often punished and actual cooperation is prohibited as bringing disturbance and unrest' (1992, page 76). In this way schools, consciously or unconsciously, stimulate an individualist attitude in pupils, who are taught that competition and rivalry are the major human values. 'Stand up for yourself' and especially 'do not share your knowledge with others', these are the implicit orientations on values children receive at school. Naturally this is a somewhat over-simplified picture. In many renewal schools, such as those based on Freinet, Jena Plan and Dalton education, learning to cooperate is part of the basic philosophy. In a number of 'regular' schools as well such an approach can be found. But for by far the majority of children and young people in present-day education the major frame of reference is the individual pursuit of certificates, which of course intensifies as the school career advances.

Such contradictions are not coincidences. They logically follow from the historical split between the acquisition of knowledge and practical experience that has characterized education for a long time. Long ago Dewey pointed out the consequences of this divergence. If there is no organic connection between the method and the substance of knowledge on the one hand and moral growth on the other, a type of knowledge comes into being that is not integrated with day-to-day practice, action and experience. In this way morality degenerates to moralism: a framework of isolated virtues (1923, page 418). This split between learning, activity and morality may be traced back to the Cartesian dichotomy of physical reality and spiritual consciousness. According to Dewey this could be breached only in an educational system in which learning is accompanied by activities with a social aim, and in which social life is used as material for learning. School should be a miniature community enabling connection between experience within and outside its walls. Cognitive, social and moral learning are thus forged together. In this way young people learn to handle knowledge and power in mutual respect. They develop a moral attitude rooted in social concern, solidarity and ability for creative adaptation in a changing society. *Learning by living*, that was what Dewey considered the essence of democratic school education. The current, rather artificial attempts to restore standards and values in an isolated form through the education system are a faint, probably ineffective reflection of this. By withholding from the pupils the opportunity to develop moral opinions and to test them against concrete social experience, education for citizenship easily acquires the character of a 'lesson in good and evil'. It is a logical and understandable consequence of a system which divorces theory and practice that many teachers complain that moral education is not part of their work. Considered in this light, Dewey's message, 70 years later, has lost little topicality.

The possibilities of participation

Experiments such as those by Dewey and Boeke, aimed as they were at reforming society itself through socializing and democratizing education, were granted only a short life. The main reason is that public support had always been lacking. The same applies to the proposals made in the Contour Memorandum to increase equal opportunities for young people through the educational system. It is hardly an accident that these social elements have never made it politically, whereas the proposals for further individualization of education gradually seem to get an ever warmer welcome. It is clearly easier to reach consensus on the latter. The possibility that the education system actually has to do something about the problems of social segregation are very much open to doubt. De Vries puts it that more equal opportunities within education must primarily be ascribed to autonomous developments outside it. In order to push back inflation of certificates, curriculum pragmatization and the effect of increasing inequality that education has, the author thinks measures are needed which not only increase employment, but promote a just division of work, income and social security (1993, page 165).

However true such an observation may be, in this way the potentials of education, and with them those of future citizens, are passed over in a few very big sociological steps. Or, to put it the other way round: relatively simple changes that are also conceivable within education can yet make a major contribution to the development of a democratic 'habitus', which in turn is a condition for a more just society. This sounds idealistic and perhaps even naïve since, as stated above, history has shown that without adequate public support significant changes are not possible. Yet there are good reasons to expect that support is growing. This is perhaps not a result of idealistic motives, but rather because of the views of young people themselves, changes in the education market and growing unrest about 'the problem of youth'.

Firstly, the Netherlands Council for Youth Policy (1992) mentions on the basis of research three dimensions which make life at school attractive for young people[9]. These are:

1 a positive social climate in which pupils have enough responsibility and room for negotiation

2 a stimulating environment for learning, in which the supply matches their needs and capabilities, and which contains sufficient steering possibilities for them

3 the presence of connections with the world outside.

---

[9]These three dimensions were drawn up on the basis of various studies into pupils' perception of their environment, including those by van der Linden and Dijkman (1989), de Vries (1987, 1988) and Matthijssen (1991).

Research into the living environment of young people between 12 and 21 years old shows that motivation and dedication to achievement at school is related to *inter alia* the possibilities the school offers for consultation and participation in decision-making (van der Linden, 1990). Both formal democracy at school (for instance the students' council), and informal democracy (are they listened to, can they participate in decision-making on things they think important) strongly influence pupils' satisfaction with the total school climate[10]. The two aspects of 'socialization' of education we mentioned before: the school as a space in which to practise commitment and the creating of connections between school and society, prove not only to be relevant from the point of view of education for citizenship, but at the same time increase the commitment to school and the motivation to learn.

Secondly, in future this could be a major argument for schools to adapt their organization in a more democratic direction. Increases in scale and mergers lead to shortage in the pupil market, and stimulate schools to stress their distinctive features. This will make the schools more inclined to be guided by the customer's wishes and requirements. Next to the level of education, the climate at school is an increasingly important motive in choosing, which means that the offer of participation will become a weapon in the struggle for pupils. Whereas now school board, management and staff often consider participation a threat to school order (Deen, 1992, page 62), it may well become a factor that will partly decide the chances of survival of a school in future.

Thirdly, the research by van der Linden shows that there is a reasonably large group of young people (12%) who have a strong dislike of school, for the very reason that they cannot in any way share in decisions there. They feel that management and staff are not at all concerned with their opinion. Notably LBO (lower secondary vocational training) pupils are strongly represented in this group. Therefore the lack of opportunities for participation could well be a major factor in connection with early drop-out, a problem that in its turn is thought to be bound up with marginalization and juvenile delinquency (Ministry of Welfare, Public Health and Cultural Affairs, WVC, 1993; Ministry of Justice, 1994)[11]. It

---

[10]Six per cent of the pupils questioned in this study were very satisfied with the possibilities for consultation at school, 82 per cent expressed average satisfaction and 12 per cent were not satisfied at all.

[11]Although the statistic connection between absenteeism and dropping out on the one hand, and delinquency on the other, has been shown several times, de Vries holds that there is no question of any causal relationship. According to him, truancy, early dropping out and vandalism or misbehaviour are consequences of the same underlying causes: the relative lack of perspective regarding the living conditions and the resulting lack of social ties of young people from the lower strata of society (ibid., page 100).

seems quite plausible that behavioural problems such as rowdyism and delinquency have a direct connection with the position of tutelage and lack of responsibility in which young people find themselves for a longer and longer period (cf. de Vries, 1993, page 70). The strengthening of their commitment to what happens at school – which for many of these youngsters may well be a first chance to have the positive feeling of being a respected member of society – may therefore be considered a contribution to the breaching of this social 'offside position' (a term Van Hessen uses, 1965). In any case it is an approach that addresses young people's potential. It is in sharp contrast to the recommendations of a national committee on juvenile delinquency, who in their report cannot get beyond a repressive approach as far as education is concerned: 'in view of the relation between chronic truancy, early drop-out and juvenile delinquency, schools are to ensure a careful registration of and checking on absenteeism, where needed, in cooperation with compulsory education officials, followed by an immediate reaction directed at parents and pupil. It should be examined in what way, through incentives and sanctions, the parents of systematic truants can be brought in to deal with this undesirable behaviour' (Ministry of Justice, 1994, pages 36–37). This is a typical 'more of the same' solution, a negative approach which will probably have as its only result that young people find new ways to duck out of this problematizing regime. For this reason also the time is ripe for research into the preventive effects of possibilities for participation in education.

The wheel of participation need not be entirely invented again. In addition to the educational experience stored up in the historical experiments mentioned, present-day education also produces sufficient successful examples to show that active participation by pupils is not just a utopia. In this respect a number of 'traditional' renewal schools, such as the Freinet schools have made most headway. Both the democratic education of pupils (through class meetings) and the cross-connections between learning at school and experiences outside (educational projects and learning by discovery) are basic elements in such schools. Group-oriented work and learning to cooperate have been quite far developed in this type of school, as in Jena Plan schools. In the last few years more and more experiments have been conducted attempting to develop learning by experience by means of cooperation between educational and other institutions (such as community centres, municipal services and enterprises) (Ministry of Education, 1992). Usually such experiments are in the context of social renewal. Cooperation between education, parents and external bodies is considered a major means to crack the marginalization and deprivation which large groups of young people are associated with. The project group believes that participation of pupils in the school and a curriculum which meshes with the pupils' perception of their environment may prevent dropping out and may raise the social perspectives of these groups.

Opportunities for active social participation of pupils therefore appear to be on the increase. Both the working of the educational market and the practice of social renewal play a part. The introduction of a new Act on participation in education and a legal obligation to draw up a pupils' charter may basically be seen as political recognition of greater personal responsibility of pupils. Practice proves, however, that many schools prefer to restrict consultation and participation in decision-making to institutions such as a pupils' parliament or a school council. Such indirect systems have very little to do with participation as a means of education for citizenship. Active commitment after all is restricted in this way to a few pupils. They will undoubtedly learn a lot, but for a large majority an annual election is the limit of their social education. Such participation in decision-making is of cosmetic rather then educational importance.

Conclusions

We have seen that a lot has changed in education, but at the same time much has remained the same. *The changes*: modern schools pay much more attention to the individual pupil, to development of his capabilities and to counselling in case of problems. The broadening of the educational supply – besides instrumentation there is more interest in orientation – is getting established in primary schools and in basic education. Moreover, an extensive system of remedial education has grown up around regular education ranging from guidance and counselling of individual pupils to an expanding network of special schools. In this sense the personalistic ideals of the Reform Movement appear to have been realized to a considerable extent. Most children in the western education system have little cause for complaint as to the individual attention they receive. It could even be posed that the so-called broadening of care is entirely in line with the orientation towards problems which has taken root in the social approach to young people (cf. Chapter 1). The imminent failure of a pupil or his dropping out sets in motion an individualizing apparatus supplying guidance, counselling, remedial teaching. If all this is not successful the pupil can be referred to special education, truancy projects or cooperative programmes run by schools and youth social work. *What has remained unchanged?*: Education is still a body that arbitrates in social selection. The 'power of the keys' in the distribution of social positions which Idenburg (1958) already attributed to the school in 1958 looks practically intact[12]. It is true that

---

[12]By the notion 'power of the keys' Idenburg meant the explicit or implicit mechanisms of selection wielded by the school, for instance the authority the school has over the pupils regarding certificates.

the educational opportunities have become less directly dependent on the parents' profession and income – the literal class character has diminished – but they are still strongly connected with their level of education (de Vries, 1993, page 156). Yet at the same time success and failure in education have been made more individual. Many teachers and social workers lay the blame for failure on the pupil himself, or on the parents who have provided insufficient school or preschool stimulation. Selection and segregation by means of schools have been excessively psychologized. For the very reason that these processes have been embedded in a framework of care, they are experienced as personal and less as an effect of the educational system. Looking at all this from the point of view of education for citizenship, one cannot but record that the school still largely provides its pupils with an individualistic image of man. Everything is about 'your' performance, to find the best place for 'you', to help 'you' with your problems. The formation of such images is not confined to education, but mirrors modern culture and society. Many parents support and stimulate this position, for quite understandable reasons for that matter. It would be an illusion to think that education of its own accord could reverse this tendency, apart from the question whether there is consensus on the matter. On the other hand we should be conscious of the consequences of such unidirectional education. Children who grow up in a community (the school) which discourages the communal, do not develop a sense of community. Those who are not taught that cooperation with, and respect for others can be a means to progress, are prepared only for running a rat race. It is difficult for a society which, by a steady lengthening of school careers, denies young people their own responsibility for ever longer periods, to reproach the young for lack of social feeling. And a school which asserts to value, and wishes to stimulate, the commitment of children but then gives them too little opportunity, undermines the confidence in the democratic quality of society at an early age. This causes the arguments for the raising of standards and values and the restoration of the educational assignment of the school to appear in a peculiar light.

Up to the present, education has mainly been a 'supply-oriented' institution. That is to say, when decisions are made about the curriculum and the organizational structure of the school, the demands of consumers, pupils and parents play a minor part. The strict regulations schools have to observe make this situation permanent. Meanwhile, it looks as if there will be some change. Schools are getting more leeway for their own policies, so that they can operate more independently, for instance in regard to staff, finance and quality of education. Schools are expected to adopt a more market- and demand-oriented position in future (Kickert & van Koolwijk, 1992). It has been found that pupils attach great value to an open, democratic atmosphere at school and a society-oriented curriculum. For this reason the chances to realize participation and social orientation at school may well be greater than in the times of Dewey, Boeke and the

Contour Memorandum. It is not really surprising that motives such as combatting deprivation and preventing dropping out make a sizeable contribution. After all, education has always been given (and has accepted) the task of averting problems manifesting themselves on the lowest rungs of society. The operation of the market and social renewal could together start a movement which might positively influence the opportunities for young people to participate in education, and in that way their active social commitment. But the operation of the market is not without its risks. If the control of education would be left entirely to the free play of market forces, a situation could arise wherein the right of the strongest parents and pupils prevail. Learning to pursue self-interest will then take the place of a type of education for citizenship which strives for democratic outlook, solidarity and a sense of social responsibility. A society which allows this calls down upon itself the consequences just described. It is in no position to reproach young people for a lack of civic sense.

References

ABOP (1989) *De bedrijvige school*. Amsterdam: ABOP.

Ahlers J (1975) *Meer mensen mondig maken*. Samenvatting van discussienota 'Contouren van een toekomstig onderwijsbestel' van het ministerie van Onderwijs en Wetenschappen. 's-Gravenhage: Staatsuitgeverij.

Bakker K, T ter Bogt & M de Waal (1993) *Opgroeien in Nederland*. Amersfoort: ACCO/NIZW.

Carpay JAM (1994) *Een school voor toekomstige burgers*. Tekst van de derde Langeveld-lezing gehouden op 20-4-1994. Utrecht: ISOR.

Damon W (1979) *The social world of the child*. San Francisco: Jossey-Bass Publishers.

Damon W (1988) *The moral child. Nurturing children's natural moral growth*. New York: The Free Press.

Dasberg L (1993) *Meelopers en dwarsliggers*. Amsterdam/Hoevelaken: Trouw & Christelijk Pedagogisch Studiecentrum.

Deen N (1992) *Mensen scholen mensen. Beschouwingen over onderwijs*. Groningen: Wolters-Noordhof.

Dewey JS (1899) *The school and society*. Gebruikt: Nederlandse vertaling 'School en Maatschappij', Groningen: J.B. Wolters, 1929.

Dewey JS (1923) *Democracy and education. An introduction to the philosophy of education*. New York: The Macmillan Company.

Diekstra RFW (1992) De adolescentie: biologische, psychologische en sociale aspecten. In: RFW Diekstra (ed) *Jeugd in ontwikkeling*. 's-Gravenhage: SDU. pp. 111–57.

Doornbos K (red) (1991) *Samen naar school. Aangepast onderwijs in gewone scholen*. Nijkerk: Intro.

Doornbos K (1994) *Voor waar het kan. Randvoorwaarden voor retentief basisonderwijs in het licht van 'Weer samen Naar School'*. Amsterdam: Instituut voor Pedagogische Wetenschappen Universiteit Amsterdam.

Graaff C de (1994) 'Weer Samen Naar School' is nog niet eens begonnen! *PCO-Magazine 3*, 22-1-94. pp. 2–4.

Gunsteren HR van ea (1992) *Eigentijds burgerschap*. Rapport van de Wetenschappelijke Raad voor het Regeringsbeleid. 's-Gravenhage: SDU.

Hessen JS van (1965) *Samen jong zijn*. Assen: Van Gorcum/Prakke.

Hofstee W (1992) *Een curriculum voor burgerschap*. zie Wetenschappelijke Raad voor het Regeringsbeleid 1992b, pp. 257–83.

Idenburg Ph J (1958) *De sleutelmacht van de school*. Groningen: Wolters.

Kerkhoff A (1989) De geschiedenis herhaalt zich: onderwijskansen van allochtone kinderen. *Migrantenstudies*, 2. pp. 32–48.

Kickert WJM & Q van Koolwijk (1992) *Onderwijs in de samenleving: een toekomstverkenning*. Enschede: SLO.

Kohlberg L (1970) Education for justice: a modern statement of the platonic view. In: JM Gustafson, RS Peters, L Kohlberg, B Bettelheim & K Keniston (eds) *Moral education, five lectures*. Cambridge, Mass: Harvard University Press.

Kuipers HJ (1992) *De wereld als werkplaats. Over de vorming van Kees Boeke en Beatrice Cadbury*. Amsterdam: IISG.

Linden FJ van der (1990) *Groot worden in een klein land. Feiten en cijfers uit het onderzoek naar de leefwereld van jongeren tussen 12 en 21 jaar*. Nijmegen: ITS.

Linden FJ van der & TA Dijkman (1989) *Jong zijn en volwassen worden in Nederland*. Nijmegen: Hoogveld Instituut.

Lockwood AL (1978) Effects of values clarification and moral development curricula on school-age subjects: a critical review of recent research. *Review of Education Research*, **48**. pp. 325–64.

Matthijssen MAJ (1991) *Lessen in orde: een onderzoek naar leerlingenperspectieven in het voortgezet onderwijs*. Amersfoort: ACCO.

Ministerie van Justitie (1994) *Met de neus op de feiten. Aanpak jeugdcriminaliteit*. Rapport opgesteld door de commissie Van Montfrans-Hartman. 's-Gravenhage: Ministerie van Justitie Directie jeugdbescherming en Reclassering.

Ministerie van Onderwijs en Wetenschappen (1990) *Weer samen naar school. Perspectief om leerlingen ook in reguliere scholen onderwijs op maat te bieden.* 's-Gravenhage.

Ministerie van Onderwijs en Wetenschappen (1992) *Zo kan het ook: voorbeelden van sociale vernieuwing in het onderwijs.* 's-Gravenhage.

Ministerie van Welzijn, Volksgezondheid en Cultuur (1993) *Jeugd verdient de toekomst. Nota intersectoraal jeugdbeleid.* 's-Gravenhage: WVC.

Mollenhauer K (1986) *Vergeten samenhang. Over cultuur en opvoeding.* Meppel: Boom.

Raad voor het Jeugdbeleid (1992) *Zin in school. Een leefbare school voor een geschakeerde jeugd.* Amsterdam: Raad voor het Jeugdbeleid.

Raths LE, M Harmin & SB Simon (1975) *Values and teaching: Working with values in the classroom.* Columbus, Ohio: C.E. Merrill.

Roland Holst H (1902) *Kapitaal en arbeid in Nederland, deel I.* Amsterdam: Soep.

Rubinstein D & C Stoneman (1970) *Education for democracy.* Harmondsworth: Penguin Books.

Schöttelndreier M (1994) De vonk van de basisvorming begint over te slaan. *Volkskrant*, 15–3. p. 11.

Teunissen F (1992) De school: méér dan een onderwijsinstelling. In: AJ Dieleman & P Span (red) *Pedagogiek van de levensloop.* Amersfoort/Heerlen: ACCO, Open Universiteit, pp. 116–30.

Vries G de (1987) *Schoolcultuur als uitdaging en opgave: over verzuim, delinquentie en de invloed van school.* Amsterdam: SCO.

Vries G de (1988) *Schoolverzuim en schooluitval in het voortgezet onderwijs.* Amsterdam: SCO.

Vries G de (1993) *Het pedagogisch regiem. Groei en grenzen van de geschoolde samenleving.* Amsterdam: Meulenhoff.

Wetenschappelijke Raad voor het Regeringsbeleid (1992a) zie van Gunsteren 1992.

Wetenschappelijke Raad voor het Regeringsbeleid (1992b) *Burgerschap in praktijken, deel 1.* 's-Gravenhage: SDU.

Wetenschappelijke Raad voor het Regeringsbeleid (1992c) *Burgerschap in praktijken, deel 2.* 's-Gravenhage: SDU.

Participation in youth care

Introduction

Western culture has the curious tendency to place young people who, for whatever reason, have problems or cause problems, in a situation that only serves to reinforce their feelings of powerlessness. Sometimes this may seem inevitable, for example when young people commit serious offences, or when they are a danger to themselves or to their environment. But even in situations such as these, reinforcing feelings of powerlessness has a counter-productive effect: if young people are to be able to function independently in society at some time in the future, it is essential that they develop a sense of being 'power-full'.

Professional youth care, a complex network of services concerned with prevention, counselling and protection is geared, wholly in line with the 'problem-orientation' described in Chapter 1, particularly to the short-comings of the client or the 'client-system'. On the basis of his or her deficiencies, the client is diagnosed and guided to a particular form of care or legal measures. The process of giving care aims to, what is officially called, 'activate the possibilities of the young person and of his educators' (Ministry of Welfare, Public Health and Cultural Affairs (WVC), & Ministry of Justice, 1993). The idea is that young people (and their parents) should be equipped to resume a 'normal' life in their own social context as quickly as possible. But in practice, this activating approach often still gets no more than lip-service. Traditionally, youth care assigns its clients a passive role. Clarijs (1993) calls this the 'I will solve this for you' attitude. Of course, all this is done with the very best of intentions. After all, it is the task of professional youth care to prevent and solve problems, and in doing so, the best possible use is made of the available expertize. The passivity of the role of the client lies not so much in the use of expertize itself, as in the context within which this is applied. It is precisely this context that often reflects the opposite of what care is actually aiming to do. In the process of being helped, for example in the case of voluntary or involuntary admission, the client loses that very independence and grip on his/her environment that the intervention is aiming to achieve; or, in the case of ambulant treatment, when a 'new' type of behaviour is being worked on while the environment of the client does not offer sufficient possibilities for putting it into practice. Here we see the same double bind that we came across earlier when discussing the participation of young people in their living environment, and of pupils in education: clients in youth care are expected to develop into competent, responsible fellow citizens in a social context that often deprives them of the possibilities for doing so. Over the past years, this problem has been gaining recognition. Various efforts are being made to strengthen the position of clients in youth care, among others, by approaching them as customers (consumers) of care, and by developing a client policy in which their position is formalized. In what follows, both options are subjected to critical scrutiny as it is questionable whether these measures actually help clients get a better grip on their own life situation.

If active participation of young people in general is a precondition for education for citizenship, as was set out above, what does this mean for young people who are confronted with problems and who have come to rely on professional help in some form or other? Is participation in such a vulnerable situation an extra burden, perhaps even too great a burden, or is it all the more necessary because active commitment can also have a preventive and curative effect? These are the questions that we will try to answer in this chapter.

Problems of youth and youth care

In the Netherlands, as in most other western countries, the social care for young people who have problems finds its origins in the nineteenth century when church and citizenry began to be seriously concerned about the social and moral dangers of criminal and neglected children. Private initiative founded various 'societies' to do something about the moral uplifting of working-class children. Thus, during the first half of that century, attempts were made to organize the supervision of poor families through a system of patronage, to improve the situation of young prisoners, and to establish colonies for orphans, foundlings, and deserted children. From 1830 onwards, a great many homes were founded, first mainly for orphans, later also for neglected and criminal children. To begin with, the authorities only concerned themselves with the latter category, for whose punishment and re-education they considered themselves responsible[1]. During the second half of the century, however, a number of measures were taken to protect children against excessive abuse. One instance is the Dutch Child Labour Act (Wet op de Kinderarbeid) which was introduced in 1874. van Nijnatten (1986) describes how such normalizing measures gradually began to support the already existing 'moralizing practices of private initiatives'. Around the turn of the century, laws were introduced that made it possible

---

[1]For an extensive review of the historical development of residential youth care during the period 1814–1914, see Dekker (1985).

to restrict parental rights[2]. The pedagogical-legal child welfare service was charged with implementing these laws. For the first time, the State was officially able to intervene in what, until then, had been the inviolable authority of the family, in this case the father. Both neglect by the parents and delinquency on the child's part could be reasons for placing a child in care and under treatment. The disciplining of dangerous children, and the concern for children in danger thus coincided more and more. The 'theory' was that these two sides of the story were connected: young people could not always be held responsible for their criminal behaviour, because this could be the result of inadequate upbringing in the family. Although, in theory, neglect and criminality were connected, in child welfare the interests of society long dominated those of the young (van Montfoort, 1994). Attention was mainly focused on 'those children who stood on the doorstep of prison or who were discharged from prison after a shorter or longer stay there' (Koekebakker, cit. Baartman, 1993, page 32). The use of the term neglect brought with it the unmistakable mark of a criminal predisposition: these were children 'whose parents, because of circumstances, had made them beg, wander around, or prostitute themselves', and who 'grew up to be good-for-nothings and eventually criminals, to which they were doomed by their idleness and lack of moral and intellectual development' (Levy, cit. Baartman, 1993, page 32). Pedagogical-legal intervention often meant that children were separated from their families. They had to be resocialized, either in families designated for this task, or in institutions 'with gentle heart and calm, but strict discipline to guide the child along proper lines' (Klootsema, 1904, page 97). 'Neglecting' families were considered harmful, not only because of the negative influence on the children, but also because they were felt to be a threat to the moral content of society as a whole. From the 1920s to the 1960s, whole families were sometimes placed under supervision by accommodating them in special housing blocks or rehabilitation centres. Re-education and social adjustment were virtually always the main goal, although the definition of the nature and cause of the problems was subject to great changes (van Wel, 1988)[3].

---

[2]Reference is to the Child Labour Act (Kinderwet) in criminal law, the Labour Act (Kinderwet) in civil law, and the General Child Protection Act (Kinderbeginselenwet), which were introduced as early as 1905. This brought young criminals and neglected children together under one legal system.

[3]Van Wel describes this shift in definitions as follows: where in the years between 1915–1935, the term *unacceptable families* was used, particularly with reference to the problems that such people caused as a result of their way of life; from 1935 to 1950 the problem was caused by *socially ill families*, the cause of their 'moral decline' was specified in terms of psychiatric categories. Between 1950 and 1965 *socially maladjusted families* were seen as stragglers, as people who could not keep up with the fast social changes after the war. In the 1960s and 1970s, the focus was on the *deprived family*; the families themselves were not so much the problem, but their socio-economic and socio-cultural backwardness. From the 1980s onward, the emphasis shifts more and more to internal problems in the family; we speak of *multi-problem families* with disorders in the patterns of communication and interaction.

The changes that have occurred with respect to the protection of young people against 'negligence' can be typified by a shift from openly moralizing disciplinary action with respect to the family to a more neutral-sounding method of transforming family members into mentally healthy, well-adjusted citizens, along social-scientific lines. Where supervision and re-education were the means of combatting the asocial family as a cesspool of vice, prevention and care for 'problem families' are gradually taking over this task. After the Second World War, more and more institutions started to concern themselves with disturbed relationships between parents and children. From that time onward, more and more scientifically trained social workers entered youth care. The role of philanthropists and volunteers from well-to-do families, who had, starting from the time of traditional poor relief, long fulfilled a key role, was gradually taken over by social workers, educationalists and psychologists, changing the content and approach of youth care. Comparative research on child welfare dossiers in the Netherlands dating from 1930 and 1975 (van Nijnatten, 1986) shows that the assessments in reports from the 1930s were highly moralizing in character, while those from 1975 were formulated on the basis of a more distant, theoretical point of view. From 1930: 'father is a weak character who hasn't had the slightest control over his son lately' (page 97). From 1975: 'because the parents have to devote a lot of attention to the youngest brother, M. is not getting enough attention' (page 109).

Youth and family problems were starting to be treated in a more scientific way, and although this can be taken as modernization that fits in with post-war developments towards democracy and emancipation, it is often said that this far from ended the patronizing attitude towards clients. From his study, van Nijnatten (ibid.) draws the conclusion that with the introduction of insights from the social sciences into child welfare the grounds for legal measures with respect to families have become shaky. Scientific insights are presented as being value-free but this is not the case: 'what is overlooked is that child welfare is a collection of institutions that propagate certain standards concerning upbringing. The standards of child welfare are not necessarily those of their clients. By taking its own truth to have general validity, child welfare conceals its ideological function' (ibid., page 164). van Wel reaches a comparable conclusion when he states: 'In families with psychological and social (as well as material) problems, the pressure that is brought to bear on them is far less manifest than it used to be. Present-day language of (voluntary) social welfare has acquired such a dominant position that the objects of (involuntary) care have adopted as their own the sociotherapeutic language and codes of conduct of social workers... Supervision from the top down has become totalitarian, that is to say – in psychological jargon – internalized' (van Wel, 1988, page 226). In short, modern youth care is a system that imparts the norms of society to clients in a subtle way, that it is acceptable to young people. Also in those cases in which help is imposed, the client is made aware of his 'need of care', 'call for help' or 'problem'.

The question now is how do such analyses compare to accepted practice of professional youth care in the 1990s? Can we speak of a new form of patronizing young clients along psychological lines? At the beginning of the 1970s, alternative youth care emphasized self-determination and autonomy as moral rights of young people, and their socially backward position. According to van Montfoort (1994), this precipitated a crisis in the established practice of child welfare. Its disciplining function, also outside alternative youth care, was brought up for discussion more frequently. In the course of the 1970s and 1980s, a significant part of youth care was withdrawn from the influence of the judiciary and was finally, in 1989, brought under the Youth Services Act (Wet op de Jeugdhulpverlening). Then a large number of the old child welfare homes were transferred to the Ministry for Welfare, Public Health and Cultural Affairs (WVC) and later, to the provincial authorities. The most important aims of the new law were to create coherence in youth care, and to improve the quality of care. A number of measures were also taken with respect to the rights of clients, as a result of which their social power was strengthened.

What does all this mean in terms of the opportunities for participation by young people within the system of youth care? This question is important if we are to assess the extent to which young clients are actually treated as fellow citizens, with all the rights, duties and responsibilities that this involves, but also (and especially) the opportunities for development. In other words, does education for citizenship have a serious role to play when young people find themselves in a, possibly serious, problem situation?

A psychosocial view of youth problems

Problem behaviour of young people must be seen as a function of the interaction between individual dispositions and the characteristics of the environment. This is a proposition to which, little by little, all professionals in youth care have come to subscribe. But what does a statement such as this mean in theory and in practice? van der Ploeg and Scholte define problem behaviour as 'behaviour that is felt or considered to be problematic by persons in the environment of the young person (parents, teachers, friends, as well as other members and representatives of society), or by the child himself' (1990, page 18). The risk of problem behaviour can be heightened by a number of environmental influences and personal traits. As examples of risk factors in the family environment, Scholte (1993, pages

63–4) mentions the presence of serious conflicts between members of the family, poor communication within the family, an insecure and unstructured educational climate, and a lack of supervision of the child. In the school environment: poor motivation, truancy, poor learning achievements, and disturbance of the relationship between the pupil and the teacher. The circle of friends constitutes a third group of possible risk factors. Association with friends who themselves present problem behaviour and spend their time in 'risk-laden leisure activities' (hanging around, gambling, alcohol and drug consumption) increase the likelihood of antisocial behaviour.

Within this so-called model, such environmental factors are considered independent variables with respect to problem behaviour. The same applies to individual traits: a lack of cognitive-emotional skills, such as weak 'ego resilience' and 'problematic ego control' heighten the risk of problematic behaviour (Scholte, ibid., page 64). The question that is central to this model is: to what extent is disturbed social and emotional development in young people (the dependent variable) related to cognitive-emotional traits and to risk factors in the educational environment (the independent variables)? There is a lot of data available on this. For example, it has been shown that there is a connection between depression, weak self-esteem, and an insecure family climate, and antisocial behaviour appears to be connected to a lack of supervision of young people in combination with a negligent affective family climate (Scholte, ibid., page 68). The connections between these factors also give an indication of the remedial educational interventions that are needed: raising the child's self-esteem, making the family climate safer, strengthening supervision, etc. According to van der Ploeg (1984) and Scholte (1993, page 69), remedial educational interventions in the case of young people with problem behaviour must be based on 'giving a description of the specific behavioural and emotional problems of the young person, and on an accurate inventory of risk-laden personality traits on the part of the young person, as well as the risk factors in the educational environment'.

What role does the client himself play in all this? On the face of it, such an approach brings to mind the classical medical model in health care, in which the patient is primarily the object of analysis and treatment. After all, within the psychosocial model, problem behaviour is defined on the basis of a prescriptive framework in which the perspectives of the client himself only partly play a role. We recall that, according to the definition of van de Ploeg and Scholte, it is *either* the environment *or* the young person that qualifies behaviour as problematic. The theoretical implication of this is that the diagnosis can be made independently of the client and his view of his environment. By way of comparison: in the previous chapter we stated that the very limited possibilities for active participation in education is the reason a considerable number of young people drop out of school early. On the basis of a psychosocial definition, we can only conclude that the young drop-out is presenting problem behaviour, because the fact that, in the eyes of the pupil, something might also be wrong with the standards of the school environment itself, does not fit into this mental framework. In youth care practice, however, the client perspective is gradually gaining recognition. The dialogue with the client about the way he sees the assessment of his or her behaviour is more often becoming the basis for the treatment programme. For example, a lot of use is made of methods to map the goals of parents and young people at the beginning of a course of treatment. This dialogue is an important way of letting the client actually feel that he or she is not an object of treatment, but is regarded as someone whose active commitment and participation is considered essential. In this way it is possible to avoid the situation in which the client in youth care receives two contradictory messages: learn to come to grips with your own life, in a situation in which other people for the greater part determine how you should go about this.

The connection between problems and participation

Earlier in this book (cf. page 60) we saw that the development of children and young people takes place within a culturally defined field: the space within which developmental processes occur is determined by the possibilities and limitations that the environment offers. Developmental psychologists associate a number of the problems that are seen in young people with a shortage of opportunities in this field for acquiring social experience. Problems in the area of identity development, moral development and social–cognitive development were seen to be related to a social context that prompts young people to adopt passive behaviour and behaviour lacking in initiative, and that isolates and/or alienates them from the day-to-day reality of adults. A lack of concrete possibilities for participation – one could say opportunities to learn through experience – can in itself be seen as a socio-cultural source of psychosocial problems in young people. Conversely, authors such as Diekstra (1992) and Heymans (1992) see active commitment as an important means of preventing such problems.

Findings from studies into factors that influence mental health point in the same direction. In the study entitled *Four dangerous intersections* (Vier Gevaarlijke Kruispunten) (Gastelaars *et al.*, 1991), the conclusion is drawn that 'social–psychiatric disorders do not only originate in the built-in impossibilities of the individual, but also in his relationship with his immediate environment, and (on a macro-level) in society as a whole'.

Consequently, one of the basic conditions for survival is, according to the authors, 'the possibility of belonging in an environment that offers sufficient common ground for personal commitment' (ibid., page 20). From this, and other studies in the field of mental health care, we can conclude that the incidence of psychosocial disorders, also in young people, can, at the very least, be reduced by the strengthening of social commitment (cf. de Ridder, 1988). The rich literature that has developed with respect to so-called 'determinants' of mental health provides us with important leads for this proposition. The way people learn to cope with events and circumstances in their lives, apart from the nature and gravity of these conditions themselves, appears to greatly influence their psychosocial well-being. Over the past years, so-called coping mechanisms have attracted a lot of interest. This concept concerns the way in which individuals handle stress. Or, to put it more precisely, 'coping refers to cognitive or behavioural attempts to master internal and/or external demands that arise from stressful interaction' (Folkman, cit. Schrameijer, 1990). Here we are considering the meaning that a person learns to ascribe to situations, and the strategies that he or she has learnt to apply to master difficulties. In both of these aspects, people appear to differ considerably from one another: physical health, a positive attitude towards life, social skills, social support and sufficient material possibilities generally contribute to an effective coping process. In coping-research, a lot of work has been done on the influence of personality traits such as hardiness, resilience and a sense of coherence. Hardiness can be described as 'a cognitive personality factor that causes situations to be perceived as being less stressful' (Bosma & Hosman, 1990, page 16). People in whom this trait is sufficiently well-developed are characterized by:

- *commitment*, i.e. they consider it meaningful to be occupied with a problem or with situational change

- *a sense of control* over one's own life situation (also called mastery or internal locus of control)

- an attitude that enables the individual to see changes in the environment as a *challenge,* a stimulus to further development.

Related to this are concepts such as *resilience* ('hardiness and flexibility in problem situations') and a *sense of coherence.* Antonovsky (1974) describes this latter trait as 'an all-pervasive, durable yet dynamic sense of trust that one's external environment is predictable and that things will most probably turn out as well as they can reasonably be expected to'. Although there are many differences of opinion about the precise workings of the relationship between such traits and mental health, it is generally assumed that an adequate style of coping increases the chance of psychosocial well-being. 'Positive' traits, attitudes and convictions in a person reinforce the quality of the coping process and thus, the well-being of that person (de

Ridder, 1994). Various studies confirm, for example, the relationship between the degree of hardiness and the occurrence of illness at a time of great stress (Schrameijer, 1990, page 138). When people have the feeling that they themselves can control circumstances and events (an internal locus of control), they seem to be more inclined to adopt an active attitude with respect to any problems that may occur. Conversely, people who have the feeling that everything in life 'happens to them' (an external locus of control) present more passive behaviour when they meet with adversity (cf. de Ridder, 1994, page 40).

How then does one acquire a 'good' style of coping, and what role does participation play in this? Individual variations in ways of coping with the environment obviously do not arise in a vacuum. As we have already said, many factors play a role in this, such as the closeness of the social support network in which people live and grow up, the emotional relationships with the parents, and in a broader sense, the 'objective' circumstances of life such as social class and educational level. Nor can it be said, in line with this observation, that psychosocial well-being constitutes a linear function of the personality traits mentioned. At the most these can be seen as factors that protect, as a buffer against negative circumstances and events in life. Both personality traits and the way in which the individual perceives his environment are subject to development. According to the accepted transactional development model individual traits and environmental variables constantly change under the influence of the others (Sameroff, 1975, 1982). From this perspective we can also assume that coping is not a static quality, but a repertoire of personal strategies that develop in the course of time, on a reciprocal basis with the environment. To come back to the above-mentioned elements of a concept such as hardiness, we can say that it is the vulnerable or injured young people particularly who should be offered opportunities for developing commitment and a sense of control over their social environment, so that they can start to see problems and difficulties as a challenge.

Various surveys that have been done over the past years on the effectiveness of prevention programmes for psychosocial problems in young people, show that the significance of interventions geared to the individual is limited. Measures that are only aimed at reinforcing individual competence and skills in dealing with problems (coping) generally appear to be insufficient. In order also to be effective in the long term they must be accompanied by interventions in the environment of the child and young person, aimed at reducing stress and facilitating social support and opportunities for participation (cf. Price et al., 1988; Bosma & Hosman, 1990). Apart from preventive effects, child and youth participation also appear to offer enormous possibilities in a *curative* sense. Research in youth care, particularly in involuntary residential care, indicates that involving young people in the planning and implementation of their own and each other's treatment can be extremely effective. Ross and McKay compare a programme in which delinquent girls with severe behaviour disorders taught each other social skills, with a programme based on classical behaviour modification (token-economy). The participation model (peer-therapist programme) won on all fronts. In this way recidivism was reduced by 90 per cent. The authors account for these results mainly by the fact that a programme of this kind appeals to the strong qualities in young people, rather than to their weaknesses. Moreover, the girls concerned attributed the results to their own efforts instead of to the coercion of professionals (Ross & McKay, 1980a,b). In the Netherlands such insights are being successfully applied more and more in the *kursushuizen* (course houses), small-scale facilities for young people with severe psychosocial and behavioural problems. Under the supervision of *kursusouders* (course parents), they gradually learn to manage the house and their treatment together (Slot *et al.*, 1993; Jagers & Slot, 1993). In this connection, Slot (1988) speaks of a 'social competence model', as contrasted with the so-called 'deficiency model' that still largely determines the way of thinking and acting in youth care. Methods based on this latter model set up a training situation in which work is done to eliminate deficiencies in social skills, on the assumption that this will positively influence behaviour in the daily living situation. Mastering a skill, however, does not necessarily mean that the skill can also be applied in different circumstances. And this is precisely what the social competence approach aims to achieve: it has to do with the extent to which a young person is capable of responding adequately in his day-to-day contacts. For this reason, Slot makes a case for treatment programmes that are community based; close contact with society facilitates the learning of the skills of daily living (1988, page 194). In this respect, the organization of the treatment setting is also very important. After all, the daily routine is the framework in which the treatment programme takes place. This living environment therefore has to be arranged in such a way that young people are, as it were, challenged to competent behaviour. According to Jagers and Slot (1993), participation in society is both the objective and the means of treatment. They point to various surveys that show that residential forms of treatment gain in effectiveness when young people are enabled to help each other gain social skills, when they are increasingly offered more joint responsibility in what happens in the home, and when the treatment programme is aligned as far as possible with tasks that are part of social life in society.

A critical analysis of the developmental environment of young people, therefore, appears to be of great importance when it is a matter of improving their psychosocial health. Consequently, in addition to interventions that are primarily oriented to the recovery of the mental apparatus, the social context that youth care itself offers its clients is of overriding importance for successful treatment. In view of the above, the active involvement of young clients in their (temporary) living environment can be expected to have considerable preventive and therapeutic value. Not treating clients as dependent objects of treatment, but involving them as active and competent subjects in (the planning of) interventions, as well as in the arrangement and management of the living situation, can also give these young people the feeling that they can master their lives. For them, education for citizenship, important as it is for all young people, has an added, recuperative value.

The relationship between the young client and the therapist

Young people who require professional help, whether as outpatients or in residential care, whether voluntarily or by court order, find themselves in a situation in which they become dependent to a greater or lesser degree on the views that social workers develop of the nature of their problems. We have already illustrated this by means of the so-called psychosocial model of youth care in which the perspective of the young client, at least theoretically, is sidelined. Although, in the literature on youth care, we regularly come across treatment goals such as 'foster the development of self-help', 'teach them to take decisions', and 'teach them to take initiatives' it is difficult to say to what extent these goals are also realized in practice. Our impression is that while such competencies do play a role within the methods used such as social skills training, they are hardly ever used as an organizational principle for the daily living environment of the client. A set-up such as that of the *Kursushuizen* in which learning to bear responsibility constitutes an explicit part of the programme, requires a very flexible and alert organization. In any case, the conditions for this do not exist in most secure residential settings according to Jagers and Slot (1993). Clarijs (1993) typifies the dominant practice with respect to family problems and problems of upbringing as prescriptive, patronizing and pedantic; the therapist tries to compensate the deficiencies encountered and reduces the qualitative and quantitative contribution of clients (parents and children) virtually to nil. According to him, this kind of attitude should be replaced by one that is aimed at activating the client. Professionals should renounce the traditional tendency to compensate by 'consistently opting for the positive values in each family and in each young person'. By placing the responsibility for the child's upbringing back with the parents, the relationship between client and therapist is altered: 'the client does not undergo treatment, but himself sets out – in consultation with the worker – the lines for a solution to his problems. The client himself draws up the agenda for care, ... and so becomes much more a client than a person in need' (ibid., pages 3,6). Although Clarijs, in this context, uses the term 'client' specifically with a view to the family as a whole, the same kind of reasoning is applied with respect to young people in difficult circumstances. This, for example, is the case in recent memoranda concerning youth policy, in which terms such as 'demand, customer and market-oriented supply' are used.

To promote the chances of young people in society and prevent dropping out, the Dutch government wants to develop an integrated package of services that, far more than has been the case until now, is to be geared to the wishes, needs and possibilities of the client (Ministry of Welfare, Public Health and Cultural Affairs (WVC), 1993; Ministry of Welfare, Public Health and Cultural Affairs (WVC) and Ministry of Justice, 1993; Derrix, 1992). In principle, there is much to be said for an approach of this kind. An offer of help in which the client continues to give direction to his own living situation has a reinforcing effect on his sense of competence and self-esteem. But this train of thought also has its limitations. For example, one may rightly ask at whose request help is to be directed (Groen & van Montfoort, 1993). After all, in youth care, we see with great regularity that the interests of minors are not the same as those of their parents. The differences in the requests cannot always be reconciled by professionals, and in a number of cases the Child Welfare Council will have to be called in to elicit action. Moreover, in child welfare cases, it is the judge, not the client who acts as the principal and initiates action (ibid., page 13). The plea to give clients of youth care 'consumer' status however, poses an even more fundamental problem. When it is said that 'the social worker has to develop a customer-oriented attitude that will make it possible to offer services and treat the customer so that he feels he is always right' (Derrix, 1992, page 32), the different positions that the client and the social worker have with respect to one another are given a wide berth. According to Van der Laan, the first thing in a social care relationship is a dialogue about 'validity claims': the client formulates a request or complaint that is to be assessed by the social worker on the basis of his professional responsibility and expertize. But even if the claims of the client are seriously investigated and discussed, situations can still arise in which the social worker can no longer agree with the analysis or solutions of the client (Hol, 1992). This is not surprising, because therapy is often no more than an attempt to change people's thoughts, attitudes and behaviour. In this process it is natural that resistance occurs on the part of the client. This is why, according to Van der Laan, the dialogue at a particular point turns into a monologue: the social worker cuts the Gordian knot. This does not necessarily involve abuse of power or unnecessary dependence, at least, not if the social worker legitimizes his choices: in the first instance to the client, but if necessary also to the professional body and society. We could also reverse the situation. A young person who encounters a social worker who treats him as a consumer ('at your service!') can hardly feel that he is being taken seriously: after all you turn to a professional for help, not to have confirmed what you have already known or thought for a long time. Looked at from this point of view, a client-oriented approach can, in an extreme situation, be seen as a denial of the educational relationship between the young client and the therapist. As Mollenhauer says: this approach propagates a non-educational attitude towards the child, an attitude that limits itself to respecting and guiding the child, and showing tolerance towards the child's feelings (1986, page 17)[4]. However important this anti-educational attitude may be, it is doubtful whether young people are served by it. Refusing to give a mature and professional reply is more likely to reinforce feelings of powerlessness, than to counter dependence. Of course, this applies all the more if children are younger. But both younger and older children, particularly if they have problems, are dependent on adults who are willing and able to take responsibility for them. A therapeutic relationship in which the young person is temporarily put into a dependent situation, therefore, cannot by definition be regarded as a form of paternalism, or suppression. At least, when this dependence has the character of an interim phase, the explicit aim of which is to educate the young person to be independent and capable of self-help. This is where the obligation of professionals to legitimize their positions with respect to young people, as Van der Laan points out, is highly relevant. In other words, they have to be able to make clear that their interventions are aimed at reinforcing social competence. Precisely for this reason it is also important that the living environment of young clients offer sufficient possibilities for participation. Then, youth care acquires for young clients a visible character of a learning and development situation. In this way, professionals can make it clear that this is a matter of 'dependent independence': an interim phase that is aimed at increasingly independent behaviour and judgement, in which the support of adults becomes (gradually) less necessary (Elbers, 1993). Mistakes can be learned from, talents are to be developed. In such a situation it is also clear to young people that they are not passive objects of treatment, but are respected as active, competent individuals whose voice and commitment is valued. For many it may well be for the first time in their lives!

Client policy

Over the past years, changing ideas on the position of the client in youth care have become apparent in the policy of government and institutions. For example, in the Dutch Youth Services Act (Wet op de Jeugdhulpverlening) mentioned above, for the first time a number of rights and procedures

---

[4]In this passage Mollenhauer rejects the anti-pedagogical movement, as expressed by Alice Miller, among others.

were laid down that are to give clients a better understanding of, and a say in the treatment process, and that make it possible for them to appeal against treatment with which they do not agree. It contains, for example, a stipulation with respect to the *right to perusal*. Clients aged 12 years and over must, in principle, be allowed to read their own records. In most cases, institutions are not allowed to give others access to the documents without the permission of the client. The law also provides for the *right of complaint*: a young person who does not agree with a certain decision can lodge a complaint with a committee that must have at least one independent member. Further to this, a separate bill is currently being prepared concerning the right to complain. It is to achieve uniformity in the regulations concerning complaints and the appointment of external complaints committees. In a number of decrees that are based on the law, the government has formulated requirements with respect to the quality of youth care. These stipulate that services are obliged to draw up a *plan of care* for each client. This plan must always be discussed with the client himself, and if circumstances permit, with his parents. *Participation in decision-making* by clients as a group is to be promoted by setting up consultancy and advisory bodies within institutions, and by stimulating the creation of client organizations[5].

What has been the effect of all these stipulations, regulations and incentives? Despite laws and regulations young people still seem to have little idea of their rights, hardly appear to look for them and make little use of their right to lodge complaints. To improve this situation, the Dutch government has decided to experiment with a system of complaints support and mediation in which independent intermediaries are called in to inform young people about their rights and, if need be, to help them submit a complaint (Ministry of Welfare, Public Health and Cultural Affairs (WVC) and Ministry of Justice, 1993). An analysis of provincial plans for youth care (NIZW, 1993a) shows that the different aspects of client policy are still not getting much attention. This applies particularly to the right to perusal, which barely gets a mention in the plans. Also the involvement of clients, parents and foster parents in the management of organizations has not yet taken off. Analysis of work plans and annual reports of institutions reveals a slightly different picture (NIZW, 1993b). From this we see that many institutions, at least on paper, attach great importance to the realization of client policy because they see this as an important means of stimulating the quality of their services. Or, as one respondent put it, 'If staff are not prepared to see the client behind the product, the chances are that the product itself will be an utter failure. This applies in trade and industry, it also applies to youth care' (ibid., page 42). The way in which this policy is

---

[5]For a further specification of stipulations and arrangements, see Tilanus, 1990, among others.

being given shape varies enormously. While most institutions are intensively occupied with improving the information that is given to clients, the nature of the information provided is, by and large, very general. The extent to which the client is actually involved in drawing up and evaluating the plan of care that the law has stipulated is not yet clear. The impression is that this is only being done sporadically. Indeed, many institutions have not yet started drawing up plans of care at all (Meijerink, 1993).

Most institutions and authorities associate the concept of client participation with public consultation and participation in decision-making. At the regional and national levels, client organizations are of practically no consequence. It is true that there are a number of action groups and parent organizations, particularly in the field of child welfare, but as yet these do not know how to join forces and exert any real influence on policy. Certainly by comparison with the 1970s when groups such as the Pressure Group of Minors were the centre of attention, young clients barely have a voice. Within institutions too, this form of client participation lies dormant. We know of only a few examples of residents' committees that function reasonably to well in residential or semi-residential institutions. These committees mostly consist of six to eight young people varying in age from ten to eighteen. As a rule they concern themselves with household and recreational matters (van Koutrik & Bluys, 1991; Huisman & Nijmeijer, 1993). However, the lack of continuity and the very narrow base of support are frequent bottlenecks in the functioning of residents' committees. By the time young people have gained enough experience with such bodies, their stay in the institution has usually ended. Besides, the contact between the representative and his supporters leaves much to be desired. Group discussions devoted to this are often given low priority by the youngsters. Here we have the Achilles heel of this form of client participation. Experience has shown that when initiatives for systems of public consultation are taken from above, as it were, to legitimize the democratic functioning of institutions, these are of little interest to young people. Student councils in schools arouse little enthusiasm if the daily reality in the classroom does not challenge the pupils to active commitment. By the same token, we cannot expect that many young clients will feel called upon to hold meetings at an abstract level about the doings of an institution (or even higher: at policy level) when there is no basis for active commitment in their own primary social group. 'I have my doubts as to whether young clients are prepared to invest time and energy in a client movement, or a residents' committee that deals with treatment plans or confidential mediators', says the coordinator of a Youth Services Advice and Complaints Office (Advies- en Klachtenburo Jeugdhulpverlening). 'They only want to talk about the food (that must be tasty), and about the group leader (who has to keep his promises), and about aggression in the group. These are the sorts of things young people tell you. This is what they get worked up about' (Groen, 1994). A remark such as this could be interpreted as criticism of young people: look how little regard they have for their interests as a group, look how egocentric they are! We could also reverse the situation: who can expect young people to bother about 'big' issues in representative bodies when, at a primary level, they do not experience others listening to their opinions, wishes and needs? This is where we pay the price for an inadequate educational view of the participation of young clients, and of client policy as a whole. Commitment is not something that is realized through proclamations by councils, by adopting regulations, or drafting bills. Commitment has to be learned, it is a thing that children and young people have to be raised to and challenged by. In youth care too, the basis for this has to be formed by continually giving them the feeling that their contribution is valued. Certainly in institutions in which young people spend a large proportion of their time, the creation of a social climate in which participation of all clients is stimulated is very important. Only when active commitment at the level of the client community is raised to a fundamental principle of care, is there any chance of creating a mature form of democracy via a system of indirect representation. Organizations or institutions which complain about a lack of interest and effort with respect to democracy on the part of clients, are misguided. They want clients to have a say in things, but they forget that they themselves have to lay the basis for this in their daily interaction with the young people who have been entrusted to their care. In principle, the same thing applies to arrangements concerning the right to perusal and the right of complaint. However important it may be to strengthen the legal position of young people, client policy that puts this first is starting at the wrong end. When a client claims his right to perusal, when complaints are lodged, this means that the dialogue between the social worker and the client has failed. Care has not succeeded in legitimizing itself in the eyes of the young person nor in gaining his confidence. Coenen and Verhaak state that putting children into homes very often does not provide the relief that it is assumed it would, but is rather a transition from a known threatening situation to an unknown, but equally threatening situation (1994, page 49). Consequently, a pedagogically inspired client policy first of all has to be directed at creating a social climate in which the young person feels safe enough to enter into a dialogue with others, and thus develop confidence in his own possibilities. In this, participation is both the means and the end.

A clear example of an approach in which participation is the basis of client policy is to be found in the 'improvement groups' (*verbetergroepen*): experiments with such groups have been conducted in a boarding house ('*Pension Zeezicht*') in Amsterdam. The aim of these groups was to improve the functioning of the organization and to make the residents socially more competent. The groups consisted of staff, volunteers and residents. 'Clients' were actively involved in improving the living and working climate. Together they discussed how *Zeezicht* policy was to be developed and put into practice, including house rules and rules of conduct. The different improvement groups tackled various 'projects': hygiene in the building, preparing a *Zeezicht* newspaper to improve internal communication, improvement of the hotel function, etc. In a report on this experiment we read 'The training in practical and social skills is thus given imperceptibly in the run of daily life. By participating in the routine of living–working–learning in the boarding house, the youngsters become familiar with the generally accepted codes of society. Policy is generally accepted because people have been made partners in the considerations that went into making that policy' (Vereniging Mans, 1992). Although this experiment concerned young people of about age 20, it would seem that the same principles could be meaningfully applied to younger clients. Of course, the procedure would have to be adapted to the level of development, but the central idea is that clients are offered the possibility of sharing in the management of their environment. This kind of active commitment is primarily relevant to residential settings. But participation can also play an important role in ambulant forms of youth care. Besides involving young people in drawing up and evaluating treatment plans, the strengthening of possibilities for participation in the various contexts in which the youngster finds himself (family, school, neighbourhood), can support social care.

Conclusions

As fellow citizens, minors have a socially embedded right to professional help when problems that they cannot handle on their own present themselves. This professional care should observe the elementary rules of democracy. The organization and implementation has to be subject to adequate social control, the legal position of clients has to be adequately provided for, and the views of the client must be heard and taken seriously. For some time now the government and institutions have been working on a client policy aimed at consolidation and formalization of these civil rights. However, this is not the only connection between youth care and education for citizenship. All children and young people, and therefore, certainly also those requiring help because of psychosocial or family problems, need a stimulating social environment that helps them develop self-respect and social competence. Active commitment teaches them to get an increasingly better grip on their own lives, to assume responsibility for themselves and for their environment. In other words: also in youth care, that is the whole network of ambulant and residential or semi-residential services concerned with the voluntary and involuntary care of young people and parents, education for citizenship is of the utmost importance. This sector is concerned with a combined educational and social aim, which is to enable young people who have problems to ultimately participate fully in social life. And so youth care is faced with a double challenge: problem-solving and education for citizenship. We have seen in this chapter that the two aspects are closely connected. Conditions which, in principle, are important for the development and education of all young people, and which can be summed up under the headings of participation and active commitment, appear to have a preventive and curative effect for young people with problems. On the basis of developmental psychological findings that were also discussed in Chapter 3, we can say that a lack of opportunities for gaining meaningful social experiences can in itself be seen as a source of psychosocial and behavioural problems in youngsters. Conversely, the increasing of opportunities for experience can reduce the chance of such problems developing. Studies in the field of mental health, 'coping research' in particular, allow us to draw comparable conclusions. Traits that can, as it were, form a buffer against negative influences of the environment and events, can considerably influence people's mental well-being. 'Hardy' individuals are characterized by, among other things, commitment and a sense of control over their own life situation. Ample opportunities for participation can positively influence the hardiness and coping style of young people. For this it is very important that the young person gets sufficient social support and has a meaningful social network. Treatment programmes that make use of 'learning by experience' confirm this. Treatment programmes that actively involve young clients in interventions and in their (residential) living environment have been proved to have a greater and more lasting effect than do programmes in which they are merely the passive object of treatment.

Nevertheless, in current youth care practice, this insight is by no means always applied. The idea that young clients contribute to their own treatment and to the daily living situation (in the case of residential care) is not generally accepted, although terms such as 'activating' and 'encouraging self-help', are frequently used, particularly in policy documents. Despite the positive experiences, forms of (partial) self-government, such as are used in the *Kursushuizen* for young people with severe behaviour disorders, are fairly rare. Where attempts at client participation have been made within youth care, so far with little success, this has taken the form of residents' committees or client organizations. One of the problems that one encounters in this type of approach is that young people are barely interested in the abstract themes that are brought forward. Moreover, as in education, the system of indirect representation does not really work, because it is difficult to motivate supporters. This is not very surprising when participation is not a habit on the 'day-to-day' level of the client community. While the frequently advocated intention to attribute to clients the role of consumers would strengthen the client's role in 'directing' his own treatment, this fails to appreciate the professional and educational responsibility of the social worker. Young people with problems are dependent on professionals who, if need be, can offer them answers. This is the essence of an educational relationship. But this is not to say that the views of the client himself should be ignored. On the contrary, these must be taken very seriously, and taking young people seriously means that response is sometimes necessary. Here again, education for citizenship and care can go hand in hand. Willingness to enter into a dialogue is an important condition for reinforcing self-respect and social competence. This dialogue takes place within a learning and development setting in which support, and sometimes leadership, by adults are indispensable. Client policy that is developed on behalf of young people, therefore, has to justify the educational character of the treatment situation. In the first instance, such policy has to create the conditions that are needed for a meaningful and just 'learning environment': a social climate in which young people can gain experience in relation to adults and their peers and consequently, perhaps for the first time in their lives, feel themselves to be wanted, valued and respected members of a community.

Strengthening the civil rights of young clients, in the vein of the UN Convention on the Rights of the Child, is a moral obligation of society. Not 'regulated', but no less essential for their future well-being, is work on the development of commitment. Participation for young people with problems is not an extra burden. It is a justified social claim and, moreover, an educational necessity. It is with this in mind that modern youth care must formulate its client policy.

References

Antonovsky A (1974) Conceptual and methodological problems in the study of resistance resources and stressfull life events. In: BS Dohrenwend & BP Dohrenwend (eds) *Stressfull life events. Their nature and effects.* New York: J Wiley & Sons.

Baartman HEM (1993) Zorgen om kinderen en zorgenkinderen; ontwikkelingen in het denken over verwaarlozing en geweld. In: PM van den Bergh, M Klomp, EJ Knorth, EM Scholte & M Smit (red) *Orthopedagogische theorie, empirisch onderzoek en jeugdhulpverlening.* Leuven-Apeldoorn: Garant. pp. 29–42.

Bosma MWM & CMH Hosman (1990) *Preventie op waarde geschat.* Nijmegen: Bêta boeken.

Clarijs R (1993) De veranderde positie van de cliënt. Een nieuwe basisfilosofie voor de jeugdhulpverlening. *Tijdschrift voor Jeugdhulpverlening en Jeugdwerk,* jrg. 5, Jan/Feb. pp. 2–10.

Coenen AWM & PM Verhaak (1994) *Vooronderzoek doelmatigheid jeugdhulpverlening.* Rapport ten behoeve van de Task-Force Jeugdhulpverlening. Leiden: Research voor Beleid.

Dekker JJH (1985) *Straffen, redden en opvoeden. Het ontstaan en de ontwikkeling van de residentiële heropvoeding in West-Europa, 1814–1914, met bijzondere aandacht voor "Nederlandsch Mettray".* Dissertatie Rijksuniversiteit Utrecht.

Derrix H (1992) De klant is koning. De cliënt als partner bij de ontwikkeling van een cliëntenbeleid. *Tijdschrift voor Jeugdhulpverlening en Jeugdwerk*, jrg. 4, nr. 12. pp. 29–34.

Diekstra RFW (1992) De adolescentie: biologische, psychologische en sociale aspecten. In: RFW Diekstra (ed) *Jeugd in ontwikkeling.* 's-Gravenhage: SDU. pp. 111–57.

Elbers EPJ (1993) De verschuivende zone tussen zorg en zelfstandigheid. Een ontwikkelingspsychologisch perspectief. In: C van Nijnatten (ed) *Kinderrechten in discussie.* Meppel: Boom. pp. 81–101.

Gastelaars MM (1991) *Vier gevaarlijke kruispunten. Een voorzet voor een geestelijk volksgezondheidsbeleid.* ism T van der Grinten, Ph Idenburg & P Schnabel. Utrecht: Centrum voor Beleid en Management.

Groen ALM & AJ van Montfoort (1993) De stem van de cliënt in de jeugdhulpverlening en de jeugdbescherming. In: ALM Groen & AJ van Montfoort (red) *Cliëntenbeleid in de jeugdhulpverlening en jeugdbescherming.* Utrecht: NIZW. pp. 5–15.

Groen ALM (red) (1994) Bundel *Werkconferentie cliëntenbeleid in jeugdhulpverlening en jeugdbescherming.* Interview met I Meijerink, coördinator Advies en Klachtenburo Jeugdhulpverlening Amsterdam. Utrecht: NIZW. pp. 32–4.

Heymans PG (1992) Moraliteit: competenties en ontwikkelingstaken. In: RFW Diekstra (ed) *Jeugd in ontwikkeling.* 's-Gravenhage: SDU. pp. 157–201.

Hol A (1992) Zakelijkheid moet niet omslaan in verzakelijking. Interview met Geert van der Laan. *Tijdschrift voor Jeugdhulpverlening en Jeugdwerk*, jrg. 4, nr. 12, pp. 41–5.

Huisman E & R Nijmeijer (1993) Bewonersparticipatie in de residentiële hulpverlening. In: ALM Groen & AJ van Montfoort (red) *Cliëntenbeleid in de jeugdhulpverlening en jeugdbescherming.* Utrecht: NIZW. pp. 65–7.

Jagers JD & NW Slot (1993) Competentievergroting door gedwongen residentiële behandeling. In: SMJ van Hekken, NW Slot, J Stolk & JW Veerman (eds) *Paedologie: wetenschap en praktijk in discussie.* Amersfoort: College Uitgevers.

Klootsema J (1904) *Misdeelde kinderen. Inleiding tot de paedagogische pathologie en therapie.* Groningen: J.B. Wolters.

Koutrik J van & R Bluys (1991) *De participatie van de cliënt in de jeugdhulpverlening.* Haarlem: Ondersteuningsinstituut Noord-Holland.

Meijerink I (1993) Ervaringen met cliëntenbeleid. In: ALM Groen & AJ van Montfoort (red) *Cliëntenbeleid in de jeugdhulpverlening en jeugdbescherming.* Utrecht: NIZW. pp. 41–50.

Ministerie van Welzijn, Volksgezondheid en Cultuur (1993) *Jeugd verdient de toekomst. Nota intersectoraal jeugdbeleid.* 's-Gravenhage: WVC.

Ministerie van Welzijn, Volksgezondheid en Cultuur en Ministerie van Justitie (1993) *Rijksplan Jeugdhulpverlening 1994–1997.* 's-Gravenhage.

Mollenhauer K (1986) *Vergeten samenhang. Over cultuur en opvoeding.* Meppel: Boom.

Montfoort AJ van (1994) *Het topje van de ijsberg. Kinderbescherming en de bestrijding van kindermishandeling in sociaal-juridisch perspectief.* Dissertatie Vrije Universiteit Amsterdam. Utrecht: SWP.

Nederlands Instituut voor Zorg en Welzijn (1993a) *Plannen in uitvoering. Analyse provinciale plannen jeugdhulpverlening 1993–1996.* Deelrapport I. Utrecht: NIZW; tweede herziene versie.

Nederlands Instituut voor Zorg en Welzijn (1993b) *Werk in uitvoering. Analyse werkplannen, jaarverslagen en interviews.* Deelrapport II. Utrecht: NIZW.

Nijnatten CHC van (1986) *Moeder Justitia en haar kinderen. De ontwikkeling van het psycho-juridisch complex in de kinderbescherming.* Dissertatie Rijsuniversiteit Utrecht. Lisse: Swets en Zeitlinger.

Ploeg JD van der (1984) Diagnostiek in het (semi)residentiële hulpverleningsveld. In: J Rispens, E Carlier & P Schoorl (red) *Diagnostiek in de hulpverlening.* Lisse: Swets & Zeitlinger. pp. 119–54.

Ploeg JD van der & FM Scholte (1990) *Lastposten of slachtoffers van de samenleving.* Rotterdam: Lemniscaat.

Price RH, EL Cowen, RP Lorion & J Ramos-McKay (1988) *14 ounces of prevention.* Washington: APA.

Ridder D de (1988) *Determinanten van psychische gezondheid. Een verkenning van de literatuur.* Utrecht: NCGV.

Ridder D de (1994) Determinanten van coping en sociale steun. In: Nationale Commissie voor Chronisch Zieken. *Coping en sociale steun voor chronisch zieken.*

Ross RR & B McKay (1980a) A study of institutional treatment programs. In:

RR Ross & P Gendreau (eds) *Effective correctional treatment*. Toronto: Butterworths. pp. 391–9.

Ross RR & B McKay (1980b) Behavioral approaches to treatment in corrections: Requiem for a panacea. In: RR Ross & P Gendreau (eds) *Effective correctional treatment*. Toronto: Butterworths. pp. 37–53.

Sameroff AJ (1975) Early influences on development: fact or fancy. *Merill Palmer Quarterly,* Vol. **21**, nr. 4. pp. 267–94.

Sameroff AJ (1982) Development and the dialectic: the need for a systems approach. In: WA Collins (ed) *The concept of development*. The Minnesota Symposia on Child Psychology; Vol. 15. Hillsdale, NJ: Erlbaum.

Scholte EM (1993) Probleemgedrag, persoonlijkheid en opvoedingsomgeving. In: PM van den Bergh, M Klomp, EJ Knorth, EM Scholte & M Smit (red) *Orthopedagogische theorie, empirisch onderzoek en jeugdhulpverlening*. Leuven-Apeldoorn: Garant. pp. 61–71.

Schrameijer F (1990) *Sociale steun. Analyse van een paradigma*. Dissertatie Universiteit Utrecht. Utrecht: NCGV.

Slot NW (1988) *Residentiële hulp voor jongeren met antisociaal gedrag*. Dissertatie Vrije Universiteit Amsterdam. Lisse: Swets & Zeitlinger.

Slot NW, JD Jagers and M Dik (1993) *Handleiding kursushuis-methodiek*. Duivendrecht: Paedologisch Instituut (zesde druk).

Tilanus CPG (1990) *Jeugdhulpverlening en de overheid*. Utrecht: SWP.

Vereniging Mans (1992) Het einde van de zachte sector? *Mans Bulletin,* jrg. **2** nr. 3, Nov. pp. 4–10.

Wel FW van (1988) *Gezinnen onder toezicht*. De stichting Volkswoningen te Utrecht 1924–1975. Amsterdam: SUA.

Building up commitment: final conclusions

Two schools

In a present-day school for secondary education, a number of pupils have complained to the school council. The toilets are always filthy, the paper is always gone, the lights are always broken and nobody ever seems to be doing anything about it. The school management take the complaints seriously and look into the matter. They conclude that the fault lies with the pupils themselves. When, in the morning, the caretaker provides new rolls of toilet paper these disappear within the hour and are then found all over the school, fully unwound. The new light bulbs often do not last longer than half a day. Parents on the school council are asked to urge their fellow parents to discuss this with their children at home. Vandalism in the bicycle shed, which has been a cause of complaint for years, seems to have come to an end now that video monitoring has been installed.

In another present-day school for secondary education, anyone walking through the school will immediately notice great differences. In some parts of the building classrooms and corridors look spotless but somewhat bare, other parts make a slightly chaotic, but very lively impression. The school is split up into seven divisions, each made up of forms one to five or six. Each division has its own place in the building and is run, as far as possible, by a dedicated team of teachers. Teachers and pupils share the responsibility for the furnishing of their division and minor repairs. Each lesson begins with a group discussion, which may be on the division's plans or problems. Not a trace of scattered toilet paper, broken light bulbs or vandalized bicycles. The school, for that matter, does not have a school council. These people try to circumvent the legal obligation to have one, because they think the way in which their school is organized is a better guarantee for commitment.

It will be clear that the two educational institutes shape their educational functions in a rather different way. Of course the former school is right in saying that the pupils are themselves responsible for the inconvenience and destruction. Clearly, however, the school does not consider strengthening the pupils' sense of responsibility to be one of its educational tasks. Indeed it opts for interventions that in fact discourage it: parents have to use their authority to restore the children's sense of values, and in the meantime the school resorts to electronic monitoring. The latter school has taken as its pedagogic basis the shared responsibility of pupils and education to this end. The importance of this is more than the absence of vandalism. Pupils gain experience in joint management of their community. The attitudes, standards and skills learned in this way could be considered part of education for citizenship.

Two neighbourhoods

A group of young people make a nuisance of themselves in a provincial suburb. Every night they meet in a bus shelter, straight opposite a row of houses where many older people live. The youngsters make a lot of noise and a mess, sometimes behaving so aggressively that some residents dare not go outside at night. Local government officials analyse the problem and conclude that the group do not have a suitable 'hangout' in the neighbourhood. The authorities ask a well-known designer to create a functional and aesthetically sound meeting place in a nearby park. In the middle of this park, on top of a hill that is clearly visible from all sides he constructs an enormous wheelbarrow made of steel tubes. On all sides it can be used to climb, sit or hang on. A splendid 'piece' with only one disadvantage: the group of young people refuse to go there. They have a few simple reasons. The bus shelter, still their favourite haunt, provides some shelter from wind and rain. Moreover, in the wheelbarrow they feel observed and watched, which is not inconceivable considering the situation. It did not occur to anyone to discuss the plan with the group beforehand. Considering young people as passive 'objects' of policy has only enriched the municipality by a costly but useless structure.

In a postwar district of another medium-sized municipality a group of teenagers also inconvenience other residents. They hang about on a little bridge and block off a much-used pedestrian route. Any criticism is met with a torrent of abuse. Elderly people and children in particular dare not come anywhere near. The council goes into action. The group of youngsters get a say in solving the problem. According to them there is no place of their own in the neighbourhood where they can meet in peace. The youngsters design a 'hang-out' made out of a high circular fence of wooden poles within which a metal container with an entrance door is placed. Subsequently the council executes the design as it stands. The place is a monstrosity: fully screened off from the outside world, always dark and therefore dangerous. Perhaps that was just what seemed exciting to the teenagers, but this is a spot where the first sexual assault seems inevitable.

Although the two forms of local youth policy were probably not made on the basis of explicit socio-pedagogic considerations, looking at them from such a perspective can indeed be enlightening. The first neighbourhood approached the young people concerned as 'objects'. Neither the question why they caused inconvenience nor possible solutions were discussed with them. The municipality simply tried to solve the problem by moving the young people on. The implicit educational messages we can deduce are: (a) your views as a young person are considered quite unimportant, and (b) problem behaviour is 'rewarded' with municipal investment. The obvious assumption is that youngsters will in their turn hardly be impressed by such a weak educator (the authorities). In neighbourhood no. 2 it was felt that participation was a suitable means to tackle problem behaviour. Clearly it was taken for granted that teenagers should already be able to judge their ideas and all the consequences independently. The adults concerned failed to put forward their own knowledge and experience. Here participation was interpreted as a full transfer of responsibility to young people. In the relationship between teenagers and adults, this amounts to a denial of educational responsibility.

Why participation of children and young people?

From previous chapters it will be clear that the care provided by western societies for children and young persons has been one-sided. These societies have a finely woven network of professional facilities to safeguard and promote the health and welfare of young people, such as Child Health Care, Youth Welfare and Youth Social Work. Educational facilities for young people have also attained a high level. Since the introduction of compulsory education and the steady lengthening of the period of schooling, opportunities for development have increased considerably. Education has also become more and more caring: an extensive pedagogic infrastructure has been created to give adequate care to pupils with problems. Looking at this scenario one cannot but conclude that the young generation has been placed on a very high pedestal. Much is invested in youth, even if only because they are now considered valuable capital becoming scarce through the de-greening of society. But this growing care is accompanied by a different approach to young people. The collective facilities realized for them are 'brokered' by various professional and policy regimes which each have their own definition of what is good for children and the young. In spite of terms such as consultation, social competence, activation and emancipation, youth is gradually being 'managed' by so many experts, policy-makers and researchers that their own young voices seem to be forgotten. This is what the examples of the two schools and the two neighbourhoods at the beginning of the chapter illustrate: we seemingly have to rediscover that serious communication with young people can be effected on matters which are important to them, and how to conduct that communication. This is of course a peculiar paradox: on the one hand a huge psycho-medical and educational apparatus has been created to guide children's individual development in the best way possible, on the other hand the limits within which this development has to take place have become stricter and stricter. Children are increasingly well taken care of, but the mental sustenance seems to become more meagre and artificial. As we have emphasized in various chapters of this book, education and socialization largely take place through 're-presentation': the possibilities for experiencing the world and life direct have gradually diminished with the growth of youthland. This has consequences for education, within and beyond the family. The direct involvement of children in social processes in the world of adults takes place at an ever later age, which forces educators to resort to abstractions. This happens in lessons at school on standards and values: pupils are expected to reach a higher level of moral reasoning through the technique of the moral dilemma, whereas their day-to-day reality in and outside school makes it almost impossible for them to gain concrete experience in this skill. Young people are denied space in which to practice and master the competences and attitudes that are required of them now and later. The problems that such a 'glasshouse' education entails are twofold. In the first place a demand for *education for citizenship* develops. How can we ask young people to meet the criteria of modern citizenship (cf. pages 27–33), if they have insufficient opportunity to gain experience? This educational demand even begins to look somewhat cynical as one realizes that youngsters gain an excess of experience in the opposite direction. Not listening to, and not actively involving young people is also to be considered a form of social education, as we have set out several times. Later we shall discuss this further. A second problem concerns the psychosocial well-being of young persons. To what extent are children's individual opportunities for development influenced by a cultural pattern in which the social demands made on them are increasingly raised on the one hand and in which a number of essential conditions for social, cognitive and moral development seem to be lacking on the other?

Conditions for development

On the basis of literature research and clinical experience Bartels and Heiner (1994) drew up a list of criteria which the environment of children and young people should meet to ensure an optimum development process. Optimum development, the authors say, will result in social competence or 'life competence': the young person commands sufficient skills to cope socially and psychologically[1]. The authors want to supply guidelines, based on these criteria, to experts in the fields of youth social work, juvenile law, prevention and youth policy. Such guidelines will enable these experts to ascertain if an environment in which a young person grows up is in his interest, and in which area intervention might be necessary. The criteria, in other words, define 'the desired characteristics of a climate for living and a way of being treated' (page 290). Specifically because they have been derived from a large number of different views, theories and studies on education and juvenile development, the criteria represent a good cross-section of present-day scientific and social patterns of thought. According to the authors, the 'optimum development environment' should meet the following conditions:

- adequate care

- secure physical environment

- continuity and stability (in living conditions, care, relations)

- interest (of carers in the personality and way of life of the young person)

- respect (carers and others should take the wishes and needs of the young person seriously)

- security, support and understanding (from at least one adult, preferably the carer)

- a supportive, flexible structure (regularity, encouragement, realistic demands and limits, room for initiative, etc.)

- emotional security (overview, structure, stability)

- adequate examples (contact with children and adults who can serve as a model for behaviour, standards and values)

- education (scope to develop talents)

- mixing with contemporaries in varied situations

- knowledge of and contact with one's own past.

What are the implications of such a list of conditions? Bartels and Heiner

---

[1]According to the authors, social competence is the result of 'the balance of demands or tasks set by environment and circumstances, and the social skills at a person's disposal'; it covers four fields, namely getting along with other people, handling material matters, handling oneself and emotional capacity (page 286). This is the sort of description that fits into a tradition of developmental psychology which strives to be non-normative. The developmental optimum after all is sought in a balance between external demands and personal capacity, without further specification as to content (cf. page 56).

see both individual and group applications. By systematically checking the various environmental aspects professional people can form an opinion on the situation in which young people grow up, they can ascertain which environmental factors require rectification or compensation and finally they can use these findings as guidelines in treatment or taking measures. Of course there is a normative snake somewhere in the grass. The assessment of the environment in which young persons grow up, even if made on the basis of general criteria, always implies a value judgement[2]. The authors are aware of this, and suggest making the assessment 'against the background of the family's subculture and socio-economic class'. As an example of this they say: 'What would be considered a normal amount of pocket money for a 10-year-old girl in an indigenous family of high socio-economic class, would be considered exorbitant for a 10-year-old Moroccan girl' (pages 290–1). Evidently general notions on culture and class can lead direct to standards enabling assessment of 'good care and education'. This is the sort of stereotype that van der Zwaard (1993) has meticulously taken apart and refuted: the education that parents (allochthonous as well as autochthonous) give is often accounted for by the demands made by their specific social context rather than by generalizing remarks on cultural background or class. Value judgements may be inherent to every involvement in education, the example demonstrates how circumspectly this has to be handled. The assessment based on ethnic or social stereotypes can itself be seen as a threatening developmental condition. This implies that it is also possible to formulate optimum development conditions on the levels of culture and society. Such collectively formulated environmental conditions are not in Bartels and Heiner's list nor, for that matter, in most other developmental psychology approaches. It is true that a criterion such as 'respect' could be interpreted as a general social condition for optimum development, but when worked out appears to be about respect in the direct relationship between the young person and his carer(s). However important such an element may be in a relational sense, this restriction to micro-level of the notion of develop-mental environment mirrors the neglect of socio-cultural conditions within the disciplines that deal with the development and education of children. According to Bronfenbrenner (1979a,b; cf. page 59) a developmental psychology which considers determinants at the meso-, exo- and macro-levels to be more or less fixed, confirms the status quo in which the young find themselves.

In other words: for those looking for possibilities to improve conditions for an optimum development of children the micro-level is not enough, they should have an 'ecological' perspective. Growing up is a dynamic process influenced by factors in the immediate vicinity, which in their turn are

---

[2]Also compare Chapter 3, pages 56–65.

controlled by social-contextual variables. The term variables is of special importance within this framework, because it indicates that these are not fixed data, but factors which can in principle be influenced. The examples on pages 145 and 146 show that educational contexts such as school and living environment contain structural elements which may check or stimulate certain aspects of the development of young people. The possibility of active commitment by young people is one such structural element. We have shown that participation enlarges the field of development, thus creating new opportunities to learn in the cognitive, social and emotional areas. Moreover participation in these areas of society has proved to be a condition for promoting social attachment and so psychosocial well-being. The possibilities for this should obviously be formulated as social-environment conditions necessary for an optimum individual development. Many of the conditions Bartels and Heiner stipulate for the primary living situation of young people can readily be translated to a social level. A development environment in which active commitment of the young is the starting point, is characterized by interest in their way of life, respect for their needs, support and understanding, room for initiative, the availability of adequate examples and scope to develop talents. As a practical application of participation these conditions may well be taken to be fundamental demands which may be made on social institutions. Social competence of young people, in other words, makes the demands mentioned not only on their direct carers, but also on the policy structuring the interaction with young people in various social domains.

Society's attention to young people

It sometimes seems that the young are a category of citizens who owe the attention given them by society mainly to the anxieties they manage to cause in politicians, policy makers and the general public: the concern for a society without standards, full of materialism, individualism and (juvenile) delinquency. The renewed discussion on the restoration of standards and values has been mentioned several times in this book. In itself this is a curious debate, since in the last few years research has shown that the largest group of young people have the same standards and values as most adults: they want good jobs, nice families and attractive houses. However, the fear of the relatively small group of young people in the margins of society is so great that it defines the image of the political and social discussion on all young people. Youth researchers, youth carers as well as the makers of policy on youth contribute greatly to this process of turning the issue into a problem. Often their priorities go hand in hand with those of public and political opinion. Research money, after all, is more readily made available for issues qualified as 'hot', and professionals and policy-makers are evidently just as susceptible to items that appeal to the anxious imagination of society. In this way youth research, youth policy and youth care narrow themselves down more and more to problem research, problem policy and the care of problem groups. A number of different explanations for this phenomenon are conceivable. Some, such as financial, institutional or professional gain, are fairly banal, but none the less valid. de Vries (1993, pages 89 ff.) illustrates this handsomely by means of the truancy problem. In the early 1980s great interest was roused in the Dutch media, several occupational groups and the authorities. Funds were made available, numerous projects started (care centres for regular truants), policy documents written and research done. Yet this sudden attention had little to do with any actual growth of the problem: dropping out and absenteeism turned out to have fallen instead of risen in the period. Not the frequency of the problem, but the social anxiety about it had increased. de Vries thinks this anxiety was a consequence of the oncoming economic recession and the attendant social tension. 'Moral entrepreneurs' such as educationalists, school attendance officials, prevention and research workers could strengthen their market position because of the picture of truancy getting out of control: 'the recession created the worried public of Members of Parliament and newspaper readers necessary to provide reception, legitimacy and money for the beneficial claims of professionals and members of the government' (ibid., page 78).

The growing influence of such 'professional regimes' on the world young people live in, and on the creation of an image of youth is connected with the shifting boundaries between youth and adulthood. On the basis of an analysis of policy reports on the young published in the Netherlands between 1945 and 1992, van Stigt (1993) concludes that admission to the adult world has been postponed ever longer. Generally studies and reports argue that postwar society is becoming more and more complex and therefore requires better preparation for adulthood. The higher the demands made by an industrialized and, later on, computerized society, the more and the longer young people have to learn to be able to function in it, thus goes the line of reasoning. Besides this however, the plea for a lengthening of the phase of youth is inspired by a virtually continuous anxiety about the moral decline or the psychological condition of young people. Sometimes this is attributed to individual shortcomings (for example in education), sometimes to social imperfections such as poor economic conditions. Reports from the 1950s[3] reflect a sombre outlook on

---

[3]Reference is made to the report *Maatschappelijke verwildering der jeugd* (*Social unruliness of youth*) (Langeveld, 1952) and the report *Moderne jeugd op haar weg naar volwassenheid* (*Modern youth on the way to maturity*) (Hoogveld Institute, 1953).

the young who are threatening to 'run wild' as a result of 'slipping out of the social and spiritual order'. Diverse measures such as family education, the strengthening of the pedagogic side of school education, the introduction of partial compulsory education and the postponement of entrance into the labour force had to ensure that society would not be ruined by selfishness and crime. In the 1960s[4] as well there were frequent pleas for postponement of adulthood (or absorption into the production process) by means of extended training up to the age of 18. In the 1970s this was intensified. In a recommendation the 'Raad voor de Jeugdvorming'[5] (Council for Youth Development) alleged that, again because of fast social changes, the adjustment process of young people had lost its naturalness. For this reason the Council pleaded for a further study into the absorption problems and mental health of young people between 10 and 25 years of age. In the 1980s and 1990s this definition of youth appears to have been consolidated. The separate treatment, notably of older youth, still regarded as a faraway ideal in the early postwar decades, now appears to have been generally accepted. The youthland pictured by Dasberg (1975) has thus become a fact. Youth has become a separate social category with a psychological dynamism entirely its own, requiring its own army of experts, policy makers and research workers. The tone of the various reports on youth, according to van Stigt (ibid., page 81), has become more and more positive and understanding. The problems young people have to contend with are understood to arise from the shortcomings of society (for instance, the lack of opportunities for development), and from the emotional tensions adolescence entails. Civilization theoreticians, such as Elias (1982) view the formation of this 'youthland' as a long-term process. Through increasing interdependence of citizens, under the influence of social change (cf. page 4) there was increasing obligation to have ever 'politer' manners. This steadily increased the distance between educated adults and children who still have to master these rules. Bridging the gap required more feeling for the typical nature of the child from the educators. The growing 'care' for children became necessary because increasing demands were made as to the degree to which young persons themselves could regulate and control their behaviour and emotions. The way in which this psychological socialization process is effected is subject to change. Certain periods show strong formalization, for instance by accentuating

---

[4]van Stigt uses the reports *Persoonsvorming bedrijfsjeugd* (Identity training young people in industry) (Ministry of Social Affairs and Public Health, 1964) and *Onderwijs en vorming tot 18 jaar* (Education and training up to the age of 18) (Ministry of Education and Science, 1967).

[5]Interim recommendation study on youth policy, Council for Youth Development (Raad voor de Jeugdvorming), 1971.

rules of conduct or by an urgent moral appeal to young people and educators. The alarming reports from the 1950s about the unruliness of mass youth as well as the plea for the restoration of standards and values witnessed in the 1990s may be regarded as such. But there are also periods with the same aim of civilising when, on the contrary, rules of conduct are eased. Wouters (1990) refers to this process as 'informalization'. When the balance of power between the various categories of citizens becomes more equal, less hierarchical conventions emerge. External compulsion becomes less acceptable within such relations and therefore heavier claims are made on self-regulation. In the 1960s, 1970s and 1980s this tendency was also manifest with regard to young people. They are stimulated to emancipation, development and personal growth, but at the same time a greater claim is made on them and their educators to steer this 'new behaviour' in the right direction. This does not always make life easier, which is why exactly in this period we see a strong increase in the supply of professional counselling.

In the past 100 years the balance of power between old and young has gradually become more democratic. The development of youthland can be seen as a process of emancipation, making the relationships between young people and adults more informal. This greater freedom for children and young people is also connected with the relaxation of manners governing interaction between adults: 'to the extent that rules of conduct between adults become easier and more informal, the discipline demanded from children and adolescents can also be eased a little', says de Vries (1993, page 143). 'Breaking the child's will', educational advice often heard in the early decades of the century, has not been an acceptable educational action for a long time. In most social environments children and young persons are negotiating partners. Parents and other educators no longer try to exact desired behaviour, but 'they are prepared to tolerate greater "wildness" in their children for a longer time, in the expectation that in the long run they will learn to handle a greater variety of situations on their own than children who grow up in the more authoritarian and formal parent–child relationships' (Wouters, 1994, page 79). Yet exactly this 'handle a greater variety of situations on their own' is at the same time the Achilles heel of youthland. For (social) education, as said before, has more and more come to resemble cultivation under glass. The increasing number of behavioural alternatives must be developed within a system that excludes young people from meaningful social experience. They have had to pay for the easing of manners and the enlargement of accepted patterns of behaviour with a platonic relationship with the outside world. The price adults pay is either anxious tension or moral indignation: is sufficient psychosocial guidance provided inside the glasshouse?; is sufficient sense of values created? For the time being this concern only leads to solutions of 'more of the same' type: more efficient guidance and talk about a higher morality[6]. The creation of more opportunities for participation, 'opening up the glasshouse' – to stick to the metaphor – should be seen as a method which may free youth as well as adults from this fruitless symbiosis.

The moral of participation by children and young people

Three critical considerations with regard to participation by children were mentioned in advance in the beginning of this book. Firstly: is the strengthening of participation by children and young people not simply a new, moralizing strategy to improve the way to socially adjust and fit them in? Secondly: is this not old wine in new bottles, because the past has witnessed many experiments with forms of self-government, advisory rights and participation in decision-making by children and young people? And thirdly: is a lot of participation not already going on within the present-day culture of negotiation? Children are already so cocksure and demanding! Is the promotion of participation in fact only a further undermining of the authority – already waning – of educators?

A new moralizing strategy?

Participation, the active commitment of children and young people to their own environment and decision-making on it, has been called in this book 'a basic right with beneficial effect'. Two arguments have been given to justify the 'basic right' character. If certain attitudes and competences are required from adult citizens, this will create the fundamental social obligation to make it possible for young people to master these skills. In a modern democracy these include the capacity to form an independent, critical opinion about responsibility, about respect for people with different opinions, about solidarity and community spirit (cf. page 30). The

---

[6]An example is the 'tough language' used by the approach to juvenile delinquency by a commission set up by the Netherlands Government (Ministry of Justice, 1994, cf. page 116). Combatting the problem of drop-outs and the attendant risk of juvenile delinquency, the only proposition produced is to strengthen registration and control. However necessary and useful this may be, such an idea is only a negative way of keeping the drop-outs in the classroom. The pattern of moral rearmament obviously does not allow for more positive possibilities, such as strengthening pupils' commitment and making the climate in the school more agreeable (cf. page 13).

acquisition of such luggage requires practice and room to gain experience. Democratic values and skills do not develop in the abstract, but have to be learned in practice. A second argument to consider participation as a basic right was stated on page 147: the psychosocial well-being of young people requires a developmental environment that satisfies the basic needs for social attachment and solidarity. These two arguments at the same time indicate the 'beneficial effect'. By giving young people a chance to make their own contribution and feel they are valued members of society or of a community, social as well as individual purposes are served.

Whichever way you look at it, however large the contribution of young people, one can always interpret participation as a strategy to fit young people in socially, as a more or less subtle technique of standardization and discipline. It is after all social education and training which are, by definition, laden with values. Anyone who is unwilling to pass on values had better not try to educate. Participation as meant here however, is also a means of developing the critical spirit of young persons. The outcome of such a participatory education may therefore well be in conflict with the values educators tried to transfer. The principle is that from an early age children and young people get the chance to experience and test in practice the values adults are trying to impart to them. Only in this way can we do justice to the ideal of citizenship.

In Chapter 2 this idea of participation as a means of education for citizenship was contrasted with two others: participation as a strategy of fitting young people in whilst ignoring their own convictions, and participation as a means of empowerment aimed at the strengthening of young people's position of power *vis-à-vis* adults. Extreme examples of the fitting-in strategy were to be found in dictatorial youth movements such as the Hitlerjugend and the Komsomol (the only youth movement allowed in the former Soviet Union). But there are less extreme versions as well in which young people are actively employed in order to realize a social objective, whereas as a subject young people were not considered to be of vital importance. In Hart's participation ladder techniques such as 'manipulation', 'decoration' and 'tokenism' are described (1992) (see page 38). In the 'empowerment approach' (Council of Europe, 1993) young people's right to actively decide is at the centre. Youth is viewed as an oppressed group in capitalist society, to be liberated by acquiring power over their own reality. In a context of real oppression and abuse of children and young persons such an approach is obvious. In this connection we mentioned the exploitation of street children in countries like Brazil and India. But in western countries as well, wherever children are insufficiently safeguarded against abuse, maltreatment and neglect, a strengthening of their legal position is called for. In the absolutist empowerment approach the importance of education and social training is however, often denied. Young people are asked to resist social evils which adults are powerless against. The active effort and guidance of like-minded and experienced citizens is then greatly needed.

The differences between these three views on participation are in degree rather than absolute. The social training approach too, incorporates elements of fitting-in and empowerment. Therefore the question whether the stimulation of participation by children and young people is a new, moralizing form of socialization, is not very relevant. Naturally a plea in this direction implies a value judgement, namely that giving an active social role to young people is important for their personal development, for their future work in society and for the development of that society itself. However plausible it is made, this is a view that can never conclusively be proven empirically. The formulation of criteria for optimum development and the direction in which society should develop, after all depend by definition on the view one holds of mankind and society. The same however applies to the dominant practice of social education that is contrary to the participation idea. Not involving children in developments in their neighbourhood, their school or other aspects of their living environment represents an implicit educational morality, namely that individual as well as community are best served by an extended youth phase characterized mainly by an accent on individual, cognitive development in an abstract learning situation. We have so much grown together with this morality however, that we hardly recognize it as such. Schuyt (1994) for instance calls 'the repression of any thought of, any discussion on, and more particularly any systematic research into the many manifest drawbacks of the one-sided achievement orientation at all levels of education' the biggest educational taboo of the time.

The plea for participation by children and young people has its anti-moralizing side. The creation of opportunities for learning by experience, 'learning by doing', gives young people the opportunity to work out their position with regard to dominant value patterns in real and practical situations. In contrast to the abstract acquisition of knowledge, this presents opportunities to try out skills, develop attitudes and test value judgements in real life situations. This is a way of learning in which social, cognitive and moral education are closely linked. In this way the transfer of standards and values is no longer learning 'a bagful of virtues' (Dasberg, 1993), but a manner of making the young discover, as much as possible, their own definitions of good and bad, in a dialogue with others, situated in social reality. To lessen as far as possible the risk of a compulsory participation morality the need for it should be discussed with young people themselves. In other words: they should be actively involved in stimulating their own participation. This is feasible by talking with them about form, content and targets of the participation. Finally, as said before, a plea for participation does not sound very credible when the young can harbour few positive expectations about their future. Anyone who sees insufficient perspective for himself in society, which is the case for a considerable group in times of (rising) juvenile unemployment and marginalization, will not be won over to the joys of social participation so easily. This is exactly the time when participation is likely to be rejected as a moralizing strategy, as mere eyewash.

Old wine in new bottles?

'One of the specific targets of youth policy is that young people are able to cooperate in their own chosen ways in shaping society and in growing up to be such adults as will be demanded by future society.' This sentence would not have been in quotation marks, if it had not come from a 25-year-old policy memorandum of the Dutch government (Ministry of Culture, Recreation and Social Work, 1969). Neither was the idea entirely new then, witness the ideas and experiments of socio-educationalists and educational reformers from the early decades of the century (cf. pages 50 and 114). Why then should it be necessary to bring participation by children and young people into the limelight again: is the rebirth of a long-gone dream advocated here? In no way has this book pretended that participation by the young is a novelty. On the contrary: many of the ideas presented here, were inspired by 'old' pedagogic reformers like Dewey, Korczak, Boeke, Freinet and others. We know that many of their pleas, initiatives and experiments did not enjoy a very long life. Nevertheless their ideas have left many traces. This is most clearly the case in education. It is true that the 'renewal schools' are still the exception to the rule of individual, achievement-oriented education, but in primary education participatory concepts can be detected (cf. Chapter 4). In fact these are 'old' reform ideals such as activating and self-steering education, the 'relationship between school and environment' and the school as a learning community. Rightly Lagerweij (1993) writes of 'the persistence of educational reform'.

The world of youth work as well has been familiar with the idea of participation for a long time. From some youth movements in the 1930s we derive notions such as autonomy and self-government, whilst the youth work of the 1960s produced terms like emancipation, activation, consultation and participation in decision-making (see page 54). After the demolition in the 1980s present-day socio-cultural work again endeavours to shape youth participation as a working principle (Council of Europe, 1993; Hazekamp et al., 1994). Youth policy in the 1970s, in which many countries advocated an active part for young people, was not very effective usually because of the lack of powerful policy instruments. In the 1980s moreover, under the influence of the general swing to the right, the idea of society being given a specific character by government policy, with youth occupying a special position, was manfully put behind us. In the new 'caring society' the responsibility for education and training was mainly returned to the family. The retreating authorities wanted to restrict their youth policy to the creation of general conditions to enable 'growing up responsibly within the existing framework of socialization'. For the rest they were willing to take only supplementary measures for groups of problem youth. In the no-nonsense era no room was left for inspired ideas on education, formative training and the future in society for young people (Elling *et al.*, 1994). Participation is returning as a theme in present-day youth policy, as is shown by the priority the Council of Europe recently gave to the subject (Council of Europe, 1994). Although the Council argues a broadly based case for strengthening the social negotiating position of young people, based on the International Convention on the Rights of the Child, the actual participation policy appears to be considered in many countries as an instrument to stem the dropping-out and marginalization of certain groups of young people (Ministry of Welfare, Public Health and Culture, 1993b).

Strengthening the active social commitment of children and young people may not in itself be a new idea, but the context in which they grow up necessitates a serious revaluation of this old ideal. In this book we have endeavoured to make clear that participation by children and young people can provide solutions to various present-day problems. Participation can offer a way out of the problem of the 'problematization' of young people. The protective youthland here seems to turn right against youth. Well meant concern for their psychological well-being and anxiety about possible derailment have made young people objects of increasing professional and policy control. This control is simultaneously the cause and the effect of a negative image of young people. Considered as a cultural phenomenon and as a developmental context it is a trend with harmful effects on young people and society. 'Committing young people' to matters that concern them within the various frameworks of socialization can counterbalance this. In this way social attention for young people is shifted to their potential. For this reason a participation policy exclusively targeted at problem groups is undesirable; such a policy reflects only the fashions of the day. Considered from the point of the requirements a future society sets for young people in terms of citizenship, participation is a *conditio sine qua non*. Participation may also help to break out of the spiral of growing demand and supply of care. A deficiency in social experience and the resultant possibilities for social bonding do after all contribute to problems in psychosocial development. This makes increased space for practising social competence a positively oriented form of prevention: preventing the problems of young people and their increasing problematization and dependence on professionals.

Assertive know-alls

> *Modern children are smart creeps who get under their parents' skins and fleece them by continually demanding new Nikes, money for expensive brand-name clothes and mountain bikes. Teachers have never had their hands as full as with this generation of assertive know-alls, who manage to fabricate a debating point in class from nothing. And the local council is getting fed up with all those action groups which, stimulated by welfare workers promoting participation, are claiming another playground. As if there are no higher priorities! When the young generation already has so much influence, how can anyone argue dry-eyed for participation of children and youngsters? And moreover: who says that children want that social responsibility, is not there a big group of young people who are interested only as far as their own individual interest is at stake?*

In addition to enthusiasm a plea for participation by children appears to stir up reactions like the above, which may regularly be heard in discussions on the subject. At the beginning of the book we already mentioned a 'smart' generation. Children know more than ever before, learn at an early date to have opinions on everything that happens in the world and do not hesitate to lecture their educators whenever they think fit. Let it be said once more at the end of our argument that this oral learning does not automatically translate into active social commitment. Participation does not equate with having a say, or following the young constantly in their needs or opinions; it does not equate with the transfer of responsibility for education and environment to children. Certainly, a children's emancipation process has taken place in the past decades. Certainly, contacts between old and young have become easier. It is highly probable this is the source of the irritation some people apparently feel when they complain scornfully about assertive young people nowadays. But the fact that the younger generation stands up for itself more and associates with adults in an easier way does not mean that their social position has become stronger. The growth of the negotiating family has indeed changed the style of authority, but has hardly increased the effective influence of young people on the world they live in. Clearly a greater social competence only does not help. Participation means gaining experience. What is essential is the creation of social and educational space in which young people, especially in the dialogue with adults and contemporaries, are given a chance to learn to weigh up interests, to take responsibility for their environment, to respect people with different ideas and other customs. This can only be learned in the concrete social reality: a reality which for young people usually exists only at a distance. Much has indeed changed in modern education. The room for negotiation for the young has increased in a relational sense, making the 'natural authority' of parents and teachers less obvious. Educational authority has to be earned and many children and young people seem to be continuously exploring the boundaries of adult tolerance. Many educators are not quite certain either and struggle with the question whether and, if so, what limits they may, can and must set to this experimenting. Thus the raising of children seems to happen within a diffuse space, the limits of which have to be decided again and again within the educational relationship. The social and cultural points of reference, previously provided by religion, birth or tradition, have to a great extent disappeared. The possibilities of making one's own choices in life have in this way considerably increased. The 'standard career' has been replaced by a 'biography of choice' (du Bois-Reymond, 1992). But this poses a problem for both educators and young people. How to prepare one's children to enable them to make the right choices, and what are the right choices? On the basis of what information and experience can a young person make an important decision, for instance when you have to select, at an ever younger age, the subjects that will determine your future (a pupil at the age of 13 or 14 at one type of secondary school).

Again we come up against the boundaries of youthland. Education at home, at school and in other frameworks of socialization has come to float in the air because the connections between youth and society have taken on an abstract character. Children are kept away from the bare facts of life for a long time. The problems and conflicts life entails are obscured for them in a romanticized form. The choice of a profession or career is not made on the basis of direct experience, for instance by spending a few days in a deadly dull office, but on the basis of an information booklet or a careers test. Views on mankind and society, standards and values are formed less in direct relationships with man and society, but are taught in artificial, psychological ways. This means that the point of reference for education and development should increasingly be looked for 'inside'. That is a hard task, which at least partly explains the interminable need of young people to explore boundaries and to engage in experimental behaviour. Moreover it makes the growing demand for professional support and individual guidance understandable. Yet the impressions with which we started this section sound too much like a one-sided reproach to the young. Of course one can imagine that some educators are disturbed by self-centred children who no longer take anything or anybody for granted. The cause for this should however, be sought in the distant, abstract relationship between youth and society rather than in the quality of the education which is supposed to produce a deficient sense of values. The gap can be closed by accepting young people as serious fellow citizens, by leading them on their way to citizenship. Making holes in youthland is not subverting but supporting education.

Conclusion: how?

'Fine theoretical talk about a dialogue with pupils, but how do you imagine doing that in a class of thirty you have to prepare for exams? A teacher doesn't have any time to spare for that!' This reaction by a teacher during a conference on the pedagogic task of teaching[7] is typical of the objections, often practical, raised against actively involving young people. In addition to the problem of time, one frequently hears in educational circles that schools 'already have so many obligations', that 'social training is not really one of the core tasks of schools' and 'I am here to pass on my professional knowledge!'. In fact the latter view is at the heart of the matter: does the teacher indeed have such an educational role? The available time after all is a derivative problem: a pedagogue from Utrecht told this particular teacher that his research had shown that the average teacher talks for some 45 minutes in a 50-minute lesson[8]. In principle therefore there is ample time for dialogue, at least if this is considered important. Comparable objections can be heard in other educational domains. Hazekamp *et al.* (1993) list series of practical problems local policy-makers envisage for the realization of the participation of young people: the culture gap between local authority bureaucracy and the experience of the pupils who are interested in quick, concrete results; young people not having sufficient skills to be able to take part in meetings and think in abstract terms; young people thinking only of themselves, etc. Finally the objection is heard in youth social work that clients are often so much at odds with themselves that active commitment to a group or institution is asking too much.

These practical objections seem to us to be mainly reactions of embarrassment. Most of today's adults grew up in a period in which it was not self-evident that young people should have a say. Professionals have been trained on the basis of a philosophy which seldom, if ever, uses the word participation. Lack of time of educators, lack of competence or motivation of young people: these are the obvious alibis adults look for so as not to have to change their educational attitudes. And perhaps that competence is indeed as yet often lacking. Where, for that matter, should youngsters have acquired it? Where should they go and get their motivation for active commitment? This indeed is the socio-pedagogical challenge: for those who want to promote the active commitment of children and young people it is not enough to record that they do not possess the required attitudes and capacities. It is indeed the responsibility of educators in the

---

[7]Conference 'What about the Pedagogues' of the (Secondary Schools Association) 'Our Secondary Education'. Tilburg, June 6, 1994.

[8]Dr W. van Werkhoven, Pedagogics Department, oral communication.

various social domains, including research workers and policy makers, to develop these attitudes and capacities. A similar argument holds good when we consider the children's level of development. Naturally it is important to attune the participation activities to this. You do not discuss cooperation with infants in day care; you create the conditions. With 8-year-olds you do not have long meetings on abstract subjects, you organize concrete activities. Equally it would attest to less than sensitive responsiveness to talk with older pupils only about the organization of a project week. They have a lot more to offer. But one significant comment should be made about this level of development. What children can handle at a certain moment in their development is not a constant factor, but is partly the result of the space for learning and experiencing offered to them. By widening the field of development, for instance by involving children from a very early age in the organization of the world they live in, their repertoire of behavioural capabilities grows. In other words: children turn out to be capable of much more than we thought possible on the basis of classical theories about stages of development, at least when they are challenged and assisted by adults.

Participation does not come automatically. It requires a different attitude from educators and professionals, it requires a review of deep-rooted concepts of education and development, and finally an acceptable perspective of the future. There is no need to repeat the importance of all this. Moreover we have pointed out a number of social developments that provide a fair wind for actively committed young people: the demand for participating citizenship, social renewal which pursues a closer commitment of citizens to their own environment and the increasing importance of young people as consumers (in living environment, education and social work).

In this book we have discussed a number of practical ways to strengthen active participation, ranging from the employment of young researchers, the managing of pupils' own divisions in school, to the setting up of children's and youth councils. It is obvious that the greatest effect will be gained, both in the short and in the long term, if participation by children and young people is achieved in as many fields of life as possible. Isolated projects make less sense, since the learning experiences gained cannot be extended and generalized. Whatever is built up in the neighbourhood, should not be discouraged at school, and vice versa. Therefore a coherent approach is called for, which is best set up at local level. The agencies, already often cooperating in neighbourhood network's youth work (education, socio-cultural youth work, community work, youth social work, police, etc.) can play an important part. The share young people themselves should have in such an approach is essential however. We should take care that their participation is not imposed on young people as intervention number such and such. How? Too little research has been done up till now (certainly in which young people are involved) to be able to determine the most effective methods of participation. In the next few years we need a broad programme, in which various forms are tried out and evaluated. A long-term programme on youth participation should aim at developing new working methods, coordination of existing and new methods, and meticulous determination of their effectiveness. This means that the effects of youth participation should be investigated from an instrumental point of view as well as from a social-pedagogic one. The instrumental point of view has to do with questions like: how can participation best be employed to attune youth policy more effectively to the issues and needs of young people?; how can youth participation best serve its preventive purpose, for instance with regard to marginalization, dropping-out and behavioural problems? Besides this, the social-pedagogic point of view concerns aspects of social integration, orientation and education for citizenship: what forms of participation by young people contribute most to the fostering of the psycho-social well-being of children and young people, and in what way can active commitment during the whole process of development be promoted? The answers to these questions are vital to strip the participation by children and young people of its possible sensitivity to trends. However, let us not shelter too much behind research. Social education is taking place all the time and everywhere. Every day parents, teachers, policy-makers and social workers experiment with it; every day creative solutions are thought up in concrete situations, without these having been researched beforehand. This is a question of common sense and creativity, from young people as well as their educators. The strengthening of active social commitment of the young people is by no means a panacea for every social problem. But it is a promising, so far ignored aspect of education and education for citizenship. If this idea gains ground, the developers of methodologies and the research workers will be able to render their services. Building up the commitment of young people merits such exertion.

References

Bartels A & H Heiner (1994) De condities voor optimale ontwikkeling. Het belang van het kind in hulpverlening, preventie en beleid. *Jeugd en Samenleving*, jrg. 24, nr. 5. pp. 282–95.

Bois-Reymond M du (1992) *Jongeren op weg naar volwassenheid*. Groningen: Wolters-Noordhoff.

Bronfenbrenner U (1979a) *The ecology of human development*. Cambridge, Mass: Harvard University Press.

Bronfenbrenner U (1979b) De experimentele ecologie van de menselijke ontwikkeling. In: W Koops & JJ van der Werff (red) *Overzicht van de ontwikkelingspsychologie*. Groningen: Wolters-Noordhof. pp. 407–23.

Council of Europe (1993) *The development of an integrated approach to youth policy planning at local level*. Strasbourg: European Steering Committee for Intergovernmental Co-Operaration in the Youth Field (CDEJ).

Council of Europe (1994) *Evolution of the role of children in family-life: participation and negotiation*. Background material from the Council of Europe. Madrid: Council of Europe.

Dasberg L (1975) *Groot brengen door klein houden als historisch verschijnsel*. Meppel: Boom. (gebruikt elfde druk 1986).

Dasberg L (1993) *Meelopers en dwarsliggers*. Amsterdam/Hoevelaken: Trouw & Christelijk Pedagogisch Studiecentrum.

Elias N (1982) *Het civilisatieproces. Sociogenetische en psychogenetische onderzoekingen*, deel 1 en 2. Utrecht: Spectrum.

Elling M, T Notten & D van Veen (1994) Terugzien voor de toekomst. Bijdrage aan de discussie over de nota intersectoraal jeugdbeleid 'Jeugd verdient de toekomst'. *Jeugd en Samenleving*, jrg. 24, nr. 6. pp. 347–58.

Hart RA (1992) *Children's participation. From tokenism to citizenship*. Florence, UNICEF Innocenti Essays nr. 4.

Hazekamp JL, J van der Gauw & J Nuijens (1993) *Jongeren doen mee aan beleid. Verslag van een onderzoek naar politieke participatie van jongeren op lokaal niveau*. 's-Gravenhage: VNG.

Hazekamp JL, VA Leenders, MAC Valkestijn & DJRB Verwer (1994) *Sociaal–cultureel jeugdwerk. Stand van zaken en perspectieven*. Utrecht: NIZW.

Hoogveld Instituut (1953) *Moderne jeugd op weg naar volwassenheid*. Nijmegen: Hoogveld Instituut.

Lagerweij N (1993) *De lange adem van onderwijsvernieuwing*. Leuven/ Apeldoorn: Garant.

Langeveld MJ ea (1952) *Maatschappelijke verwildering der jeugd. Rapport betreffende het onderzoek naar de geestesgesteldheid van de massajeugd*. 's-Gravenhage: Staatsuitgeverij.

Ministerie van Cultuur, Recreatie en Maatschappelijk Werk (1969) *Nota jeugdbeleid*. 's-Gravenhage: Staatsuitgeverij.

Ministerie van Onderwijs en Wetenschappen (1967) *Onderwijs en vorming tot 18 jaar*. 's-Gravenhage.

Ministerie van Onderwijs en Wetenschappen (1969) *Rapport Commissie Vorming en onderwijs leerplichtvrije jeugd*. 's-Gravenhage.

Ministerie van Sociale Zaken en Volksgezondheid (1964) *Eindrapport van de Commissie voor het onderzoek naar de jeugd in bedrijven.* 's-Gravenhage.

Ministerie van Welzijn, Volksgezondheid en Cultuur (1993) *Jeugd betrekken. Een notitie over jeugdparticipatie.* Bijlage bij 'Jeugd verdient de Toekomst. Nota intersectoraal jeugdbeleid'. 's-Gravenhage: WVC.

Schuyt K (1994) Het pedagogisch taboe. *Volkskrant,* 6-6-1994.

Stigt WE van (1993) *Tot waarlijk volwassen mensen. Jeugd en deugd in overheidsrapporten 1945–1992.* Doktoraalscriptie sociologie Universiteit van Amsterdam.

Vries G de (1993) *Het pedagogisch regiem. Groei en grenzen van de geschoolde samenleving.* Amsterdam: Meulenhoff.

Wouters C (1990) *Van Minnen en Sterven. Informalisering van omgangsvormen rond seks en dood.* Amsterdam: Bert Bakker. Dissertatie Universiteit van Amsterdam.

Wouters C (1994) Interdisciplinariteit als symptoom van integratieprocessen. In: L Hagendoorn, A Komter & R Maier (red) *Samenhang der sociale wetenschappen. Beloften en problemen van een interdisciplinaire werkwijze.* Houten/Zaventem: Bohn Stafleu Van Loghum, pp. 71–94.

Zwaard JA van der (1993) *El Mizan. Wijkverpleegkundigen over opvoeding in allochtone huishoudens.* Dissertatie Universiteit Utrecht. Amsterdam: SUA.

Index

autism 12

behaviour theory 57
Boeke, Kees 54
Bowlby, John 60
Butterflies Project 40

Cadbury, Beatrice 54
care aspects
   care-ethics 33
   as a school subject 30, 109
   youth care 123–44
Centres for Urban Studies 92
child labour 48
   street children 40–1, 156
Child Study Movement 57, 58
citizenship 27–33
   in education system 98–100, 109–14
civil rights of children, 30
The Competent Infant (1973) 60
complaints procedures in youth care
   136
Convention on the Rights of the
   Child 33–5, 159
coping strategies 130–33, 140
Council of Europe 26, 27, 92, 159
crime/delinquency *see* juvenile
   delinquency

development disorder screening 10,
   15–17
developmental psychology 55–65
   optimum development 148–51
Dewey, John 57, 107
Donaldson, M 62

education and schooling 97–122
   British primary schools 92
   care studies 30
   case studies 145–6
   citizenship and 98–100, 109–14

historical aspects 6–8, 48–55, 100–
   2, 105–6, 158
participation in 25, 97–122
role of teacher 162
school risk factors 128
sex education 39
social education 50–5, 79–80, 99,
   104, 110
truancy problem 116–17, 152
The Enlightenment 48–9, 50–1, 53n
ethnic minorities
   as at-risk group 11, 12, 36
   education system and 102
   unemployment and 11, 18

families 65–9
   family risk factors 127–8
   family therapy 133–4
   historical aspects 4–5
   problem families 125–6
   see also parents and parenting
football hooliganism 89–90
France 85
Freinet schools 117
Freud, Sigmund 58

Gesell, A 57
Guatemala 35n

Hall, Stanley 57
Health for All Programme (WHO)
   17
health care
   patients' associations 29
   social participation in 25
historical aspects 4–15, 48–55
   developmental psychology 56–60
   education system 6–8, 48–55, 100–
     2, 105–6, 158
   growth of youthland 151–5
   problem youth 124–7